CW00502353

VEGAN KETO DIET 2021

A Beginner Guide For A 100% Plant-Based Ketogenic Diet To Burn Fat, with Delicious Low-Carb Recipes, to Nourish Your Mind and Promote Weight Loss Naturally!

Richard Tillcot

Table of Contents

DESCRIPTION 17

INTRODUCTION TO VEGANISM 18

THE HISTORY 21

BENEFITS OF THE KETOGENIC 23

WHY GO, VEGAN? 31

HOW THE KETOGENIC DIET WORKS 36

KETO DIET BASICS FOR VEGAN 39

HOW TO GET STARTED ON A HEALTHY KETOGENIC DIET 44

What You Need to Know Before Starting A Ketogenic Diet

Steps before getting started

HEALTH BENEFITS OF KETO VEGAN DIET 54

Improved Digestion:

Healthier Skin

More Energy:

Protection against Genetic Diseases:

Protection against Cancer:

KETO SIDE EFFECTS 57

There are two main reasons why keto flu occurs:

WHAT TO EAT ON A VEGAN KETO DIET 62

WHAT NOT TO EAT ON A VEGAN KETO DIET 66

IS IT RIGHT FOR YOU? 68
Pregnant or Nursing .
Medication-Caused Hypoglycemia
Diabetes or Blood Sugar Problems
Other Medications
Underweight or Nutrient Deficient
Children .
Kidney Disease or Stones
Gallstones or Gall Bladder Removal
Enzyme Deficiency or Defect
.
KETOGENIC DIET TIPS 77
How easy is it to follow the Ketogenic Diet?
1. Be Patient - It takes time to lose weight
2. Get Enough Sleep:
3. Clean Your Kitchen Cupboards:
4. Hydrate Well - drink lots of water:
5. Look for a Partner:
6. Weigh Yourself Every Other Week

DIFFICULTIES THAT ARISE DURING THE DIET 81
Induction (Keto) Flu
Leg Cramps
Constipation
Bad Breath
Increased Heart Rate
Reduction in Physical Performance
Temporary Loss of Hair
Elevated Cholesterol
Low-Carb and Alcohol Intolerance
Period Changes
1) You probably never entered ketosis
2) You're consuming more proteins than necessary
3) You're probably missing hidden carb sources
4) High daily calorie intake
#1: Eating lots of Fatty Foods makes you Fat

#2: The diet won't be sustained since it's deficient in some vitamins and minerals
#3: As long as you keep your carb levels low, you can eat as much protein
#4: The ketogenic diet causes electrolyte deficiency and dehydration

BREAKFAST **98**
01. Astonishing Vegan Hemp Seed Yogurt
Ingredients
Directions:
Nutrition Values:
02. Sensual Portobello Mushrooms
Ingredients:
Directions:
Nutrition Values:
03. Surprisingly Keto Tomato Tart
Ingredients
For Crust
For Filling
Directions:
Nutrition Values:
04. Kalamata Olive Tapenade
Ingredients:
Directions:
Nutrition Values:
05. Silly Scallion Pancakes
Ingredients
For Cakes
For Sauce
Directions:
Nutrition Values:
06. The Keto Crack Slaw
Ingredients

Directions:
Nutrition Values:
07. Feisty Grilled Artichokes
Ingredients:
Directions:
Nutrition Values:
08. The Thundering Cinnamon Chocolate Smoothie
Ingredients
Directions:
Nutrition Values:
09. Vegan Enchilada Macaroni
Ingredients
For Sauce
Directions:
Nutrition Values:
10. Squash Salad for the Green Lovers!
Ingredients:
Directions:
Nutrition Values:
11. Pumpkin Pecan Oatmeal
Ingredients:
Directions:
Nutrition Value
12. Tasty Breakfast Burrito
Ingredients:
Directions:
Nutrition Value
13. Healthy Steel Cut Oats
Ingredients:
Directions:
Nutrition Value:
14. Breakfast Tofu Casserole
Ingredients:
Directions:
Nutrition Value
15. Carrot Oatmeal

Ingredients:
Directions:
Nutrition Value
16. Delicious Vegan Scramble
Ingredients:
Directions:
Nutrition Value
17. Blueberries Oatmeal
Ingredients:
Directions:
Nutrition Value:
18. Sweet Apple And Pears Breakfast
Ingredients:
Directions:
Nutrition Value
19. Almond Butter Oatmeal
Ingredients:
Directions:
Nutrition Value:
20. Banana Oatmeal
Ingredients:
Directions:
Nutrition Value
21. Delicious Vegan Frittata
Ingredients:
Directions:
Nutrition Value:
22. Apple Granola
Ingredients:
Directions:
Nutrition Value
23. Carrot And Zucchini Oatmeal
Ingredients:
Directions:
Nutrition Value
24. Cranberry Breakfast Quinoa

Ingredients:
Directions:
25. Delicious Quinoa And Oats
Ingredients:
Directions:
Nutrition Value
26. Breakfast Chia Pudding
Ingredients:
Directions:
Nutrition Value

MAINS **143**
27. Stinky Roasted Garlic
Ingredients
Directions
Nutrition Value
28. The Crazy Tofu Bok Choy Salad
Ingredients
Oven Baked Tofu
Bok Choy Salad
Directions
Nutrition Values:
29. A Spicy Red Coconut Curry for Keto Vegans
Ingredients
Special Sauce
Directions
Nutrition Values:
30. Quick and Easy Caesar Salad
Ingredients
Directions
Nutrition Values:
31. Creamy Roasted Pepper Soup
Ingredients
Directions

Nutrition Values:
32. Spiralized Asian Zucchini Salad
Ingredients
Directions
Nutrition Values:
33. Forever Together Courgette Salad
Ingredients
Directions:
Nutrition Values:
34. Roasted Cauliflower Soup
Ingredients
Directions
Nutrition Value
35. Fine Vegan Pad Thai of Very Low Carb
Ingredients
Directions
Nutrition Values:
36. Vegan White Pizza
Ingredients:
Directions:
Nutrition Value
37. Mini Vegan Shephard's Pie
Ingredients:
Directions:
Nutrition Value
38. Mushroom Pasta
Ingredients:
Directions:
Nutrition Value
39. Basil Risotto
Ingredients:
Directions:
Nutrition Value
40. Vegan Cheese and Asparagus Pasta
Ingredients:
Directions:

Nutrition Value
41. Carrot and Sweet Potato Medley
Ingredients:
Directions:
Nutrition Value
42. Pesto Farfale
Ingredients:
Directions:
Nutrition Value
43. Mexican Rice Casserole
Ingredients:
Directions:
Nutrition Value
44. Warm Collard Salad
Ingredients
Directions
Nutrition Value
45. Fried Broccoli Salad with Tempeh and Cranberries
Ingredients
Directions
Nutrition Value
46. Tangy Nutty Brussel Sprout Salad
Ingredients
Directions
Nutrition Value

ENTREES **182**
47. Tomato Cream Soup with Basil
Ingredients
Directions
Nutrition Value
48. Vegan Coconut Green Soup
Ingredients
Directions

Nutrition Value
49. Hearty Vegetable Soup
Ingredients
Directions
Nutrition Value
50. Vegan Cream Soup with Avocado & Zucchini 227 Ingredients
Directions
Nutrition Value
51. Mediterranean Artichoke & Red Onion Salad 228 Ingredients
Directions
Nutrition Value
52. Fresh Avocado-Cucumber Soup
Ingredients
Directions
Nutrition Value
53. Almond Parsnip Soup
Ingredients
Directions
Nutrition Value
54. Sauteed Spinach with Spicy Tofu
Ingredients
Directions
Nutrition Value
55. Cauliflower & Celery Bisque
Ingredients
Directions
Nutrition Value
56. Crunchy Rosemary Almonds
Ingredients:
Directions:
Nutrition Value
57. Simple Cauliflower Popcorn
Ingredients:
Directions:
Nutrition Value
58. Healthy Avocado Fries

Ingredients:
Directions:
Nutrition Value
59. Baked Onion Rings
Ingredients:
Directions:
Nutrition Value
60. Easy Brussels sprouts Chips
Ingredients:
Directions:
Nutrition Value
61. Crispy Apple Chips
Ingredients:
Nutrition Value
62. Zucchini Chips
Ingredients:
Directions:
Nutrition Value
63. Crisp Radish Chips
Ingredients:
Directions:
Nutrition Value
64. Fried Parsnip Chips
Ingredients:
Directions:
Nutrition Value
65. Spicy Roasted Nuts
Ingredients:
Directions:
Nutrition Value

SOUPS AND SALADS **212**
66. Greek-Style Salad
Ingredients

For Sunflower Seed Dressing:
For the salad
Directions
67. Moroccan Carrot Salad With Harissa
Ingredients
Directions
68. Warm Savoy Cabbage Slaw
Ingredients
Directions
69. Taco Salad Boats
Ingredients
Directions
70. Cauliflower Salad With Pecans
Ingredients
Directions
71. Crunchy Broccoli Salad
Ingredients
Directions
72. Kale Salad With Crispy Tofu Cubes
Ingredients
Directions
73. Cucumber And Zucchini Ribbon Salad
Ingredients
Directions
74. Crazy Asian Zucchini Salad
Nutrition Value
Ingredients:
Direction:
75. Iconic Creamy Kale Salad
Nutrition Value
Ingredients:
Toppings:
Direction:
76. Tasty Corn & Avocado Salad
Nutrition Value
Ingredients:

Salad:
Dressing:
Direction:
77. Coolest Arugula & Blueberry Salad
Nutrition Value
Ingredients:
Direction:
78. Fantastic Clean Avocado Salad with Cilantro:
Nutrition Value
Ingredients:
Direction:
79. Curious Courgette Salad with Herbed Vinaigrette
Nutrition Value
Ingredients:
Direction:
80. Keto Red Curry
Ingredients:
Directions:
Nutrition Value
81. Kale Soup
Ingredients:
Directions:
Nutrition Value
82. Creamy Jalapeno Soup
Ingredients:
Directions:
Nutrition Value
83. Chinese Chili Soup
Ingredients:
Directions:
Nutrition Value
84. Mushroom Soup
Ingredients:
Directions:
Nutrition Value
85. Vietnamese-Style Vegetable Soup

Ingredients:
Directions:
Nutrition Value
86. Green Chili Soup
Ingredients:
Directions:
Nutrition Value
87. Vegetarian Red Chili
Ingredients:
Directions:
Nutrition Value
88. Vegetarian Green Chili
Ingredients:
Directions:
Nutrition Value
89. Tortilla Soup
Ingredients:
Directions:
Nutrition Value
90. Keto Vegetable Soup
Ingredients:
Directions:
Nutrition Value
91. Keto Cabbage Soup
Ingredients:
Directions:
Nutrition Value

CONCLUSION **259**

DESCRIPTION

Veganism is more than a diet for the individuals who chose to eat free of animal products—it often involves tough decisions, difficult restraints, and more changes than just "what not to eat." Big lifestyle changes are not at all uncommon for vegans who recognize the health benefits, and environmental benefits, of refusing to support the animal farming industry. Though you don't need to have begun your vegan journey for the sake of the animals, your commitment to the eating hormone, steroid, and antibiotic-free meat supports a stronger farming industry that's more focused on plant production. No matter what nutritional value that you can find in meats and dairy, you'll always be able to find a natural source of the same proteins, fats, and sustainable Carbs in plants. Moreover, most of the time, these sources are purer and less likely to be processed and turned into saturated fats.

This guide focuses on enlightening you on the keto vegan diet starting from the basics, history, how to this diet works, what to eat and what not to eat, the challenges of partaking in this diet and the recipes for you! You do not want to miss out on the amazing benefits of this diet. Now, get your apron ready and get ready to start cooking these yummy dishes that will bring back food to the soul of your home.

Happy reading!!!!

INTRODUCTION TO VEGANISM

A vegan is a basically a vegetarian whose diet excludes meat, eggs, dairy products & all other animal by-products. In brief, a vegan is a very moody vegetarian. Basically, being a vegan really means taking the vegetarian diet to another level & also discovering new ways to keep away from products that involved suffrage to animals. Your diet should no longer be about just simply avoiding some types of food but being a relatively conscious consumer that also objects to the moral & exploitative nature of the society. For example, a vegan will strongly object to the consumption of gummy bears, because they are actually made from gelatin, which prepared by the cooking of pigskin, bone, cow skin, & cartilage. Also, some producers might add gelatin for added thickness to their yogurts & candy, & a vegan will perhaps always do their research far in advance.

Veganism has a huge impact on the Earth. Think about your favorite grocery store. What does the produce section look like compared to the refrigerated deli meats? Animal products require an astronomical amount of packaging to keep them fresh, as do many dairy products and processed grains. As a vegan, you'll start your journey on the Keto diet with a clean lifestyle in every aspect, and you won't just notice the difference when it comes to following the eating restrictions. Vegans are often used to preparing their own meals to take their nutrition on-the-go and oftentimes already have a medicine cabinet full of Keto-friendly supplements. Your vegan lifestyle has already warmed you up to be more in-tune with your body and what it needs—as compared to most individuals starting out a Ketogenic diet. You'll be able to understand better why the Keto diet works, how the Keto diet works, and how to make Keto work best for you. The Ketogenic diet aims to reinvent your lifestyle for the better—and if you're already used to the dedication that it takes to make a vegan diet possible, you're prepared to take the plunge. However, you might be wondering what a plunge into Keto looks like. The Keto diet might seem like the new kid on the block, but eating a diet high in healthy fats and low in sugary Carbs has been helping people shape up their habits and shape up their bodies for longer than you know. Why? It's because it's science.

THE HISTORY

The ketogenic diet traces its roots to the treatment of epilepsy. Surprisingly this goes all the way back to 500 BC when ancient Greeks observed that fasting or eating a ketogenic diet helped reduce epileptic seizures. In modern times, the ketogenic diet was reintroduced in the practice of medicine to treat children with epilepsy. In 1921, a scientist named Rollin Woodyatt discovered that the liver made ketone bodies during starvation or when the patient was following a high fat, low carbohydrate diet.

Research into the keto diet stalled until the 1960s, when scientists discovered that a certain class of fats called medium chain triglycerides (MCTs) were readily transported to the liver and made into ketone bodies, faster than normal fats (coconut oil is an example). It was also found that the body could go into a state of ketosis eating more protein when large amounts of MCTs were consumed.

In the early 1970s, a cardiologist named Robert Atkins

proposed his own version of a ketogenic diet called the Atkins diet, which has been immensely popular. The Atkins diet has more relaxed standards that keto, allowing adherents to follow very strict carbohydrate consumption for the first two weeks during an "induction phase." After this, the number of Carbs consumed can be slightly increased.

From there, research on ketogenic diets stalled again. However, in the past years, there has been an explosion of interest in the diet.

BENEFITS OF THE KETOGENIC

I am not the only one singing the benefits of the Keto diet. Apart from the primary benefit of easy weight loss, there are other significant benefits that you will experience as well.

1. Enhanced weight loss - On average, a dieter can lose anywhere from 10-25 pounds while on a Keto diet. If you don't believe me (and you are right, you shouldn't. Your mama told you not to trust strangers), the data is there to back up the claims. According to studies printed in NCBI and The American Journal of Physiology, dieters following the low-carb principles lose significant weight in the first one or two weeks of starting the diet. The diet was effective up to six months as well, provided the dieter followed diet principles to the tee.

2. Manage Hunger – Hunger pangs were literally absent in 90% of dieters. Although the exact

mechanism of action is unknown, researchers noted that 90% of dieters experienced a fall in hunger pangs and carb cravings when their bodies entered ketosis. A small percentage still had cravings, but a modified keto diet called the Cyclical Keto diet seemed to help these dieters considerably.

3. Effortless maintenance of optimal weight – Users have noted that they stop feeling hungry after starting the keto diet. If you aren't hungry, you aren't going to be binging on food, and this means you maintain your diet. Yay!

4. Stored body fat as fuel – If you have a jelly belly, you are one of the persons who will definitely benefit from a keto diet. Research shows that stored fat in the abdominal area (called visceral fat) is responsible for causing chronic health conditions. Visceral fat also lodges around organs and under the skin causing inflammation, insulin resistance and diabetes, and metabolic dysfunction. Low-carb diets like

the keto diet force the body into yanking out that stored fat and using it to make energy. Not only do you lose more fat, but you actually lose if from those annoying areas like your hips, belly, and buttocks. Yes!!!

5. Faster recovery from exercise – Due to the increased protein content in your diet, users have noted a faster recovery from exercise-induced injuries. Moreover, due to the higher fat and protein content in your diet, you feel better and recover faster after intense workouts.

6. Reduces and regulates levels of insulin – If you are a pre-diabetic (parents with diabetes) or in metabolic syndrome, you will benefit from a high-protein diet. Think about it; when you eat carbs, they are converted to sugar. The sugar enters your blood and raises your blood sugar levels. As blood sugar levels are high, your pancreas is poked to produce more insulin. For people who are healthy, the pancreas can produce enough insulin to pull sugar into body

cells. But for overweight individuals, the amount of insulin produced is insufficient. As a result, more sugar floating in blood and BAM...you have diabetes. With a low-carb diet, you are actually bypassing this entire process and ensuring that your blood sugar is under control. Diabetics following a high-protein diet have actually reported a 50% decrease in the insulin injection does and oral medication. Of course, do consult your doctor before starting this diet, but the research underlying this is solid. Check it out here.

7. Improved cholesterol markers – Suffer from high cholesterol levels, do you? Surprisingly, the keto diet seems to help with that as well. High cholesterol levels are primarily triglycerides, which are nothing but fat bubbles in the blood. Interestingly enough, a high carb diet is responsible for causing high cholesterol levels. So...cutting out carbs seems to have a really good effect on your blood triglyceride. Lower

cholesterol levels also mean better heart health and lower blood pressure levels. And happily, a low-carb diet also seems to boost your good cholesterol or HDL levels.Simply put, a happy heart means a longer life.

8. Improved blood pressure readings – That makes sense right. When your blood cholesterol levels go down, and your blood sugar levels get corrected, it's less work on your heart. Less work means that your heart does not have to pump all that hard. Good blood pressure levels are a bonus.

9. 9.Keto treats metabolic syndrome – Metabolic syndrome is something to watch out for, and it refers to a collection of symptoms. If you have abdominal obesity, elevated blood pressure, elevated fasting blood sugar levels, high triglyceride levels, and low HDL levels; you are a prime candidate for diabetes, atherosclerosis and a future candidate for heart attacks and strokes. The good news is that all these

symptoms improve with a low-carb, high protein keto diet.

10. Keto helps with epilepsy – The science is solid. We don't know how it works, but it works. Almost 90% of epileptics feel better while on a low-carb diet. Attacks reduce, and patients can lead a normal, low-medication life. When you consider how scary epilepsy is for the individual and his/her family, you'll realize just how much of a godsend this diet is. Read Charlie's Story and his struggle with epilepsy here.

11. Improves fatty liver disease – Fatty liver disease is actually controllable with a keto diet. The diet cuts down on all high fructose foods, all refined polyunsaturated vegetable oils, and carbs. The result; A healthier liver.

12. More Energy and Better Sleep – The common understanding is that the brain requires sugar to work, and it is true. On the keto diet, your sugar intake is restricted. Moreover, carbs (the most

common source of sugar) are restricted. This means you should be sluggish and tired, right? Wrong, the human body is incredibly adaptable. To meet the sugar shortfall, the liver modifies proteins to sugar. Not only do you feel better and sleep better, but you also feel energetic and healthy.

13. Enhanced mood – People following a high-carb diet usually report mental fogginess and sleepiness after a high-carb meal. However, keto-diets are low in carbs and dieters have reported better moods, more alertness, and overall clearer thinking. And of course, the brain is 60% fat by weight. It just stands to reason that more fat will only make it work better. Apart from general alertness, a high-fat diet also seems to help with mood diseases like autism, bipolar, depression, etc.

14. Improved digestion – Irritable Bowel Syndrome is one of the most common idiopathic (cause unknown) conditions affecting people in

developed countries. The condition is characterized by constipation, diarrhea, cramps, bloating, gas, and a range of other irritating symptoms that have no cure. A low-carb, high-fat diet seems to help considerably in controlling these changes, and people have reported better digestion.

15. Improved blood profile – By switching over to the Keto diet, your overall health improves. Blood tests for Keto dieters reflect lower levels of C-reactive proteins and HBA1C. Both of these are markers for chronic health conditions. Lower these levels, and improve your overall health.

There is a ton of evidence, and all of it adds up to show that a low-carb, high-fat diet can actually improve your health. Apart from the health benefits, it also seems to reduce weight, make you trim and energetic, and ensure that you are far more healthy.

All in all, a win-win kind of diet, right?

WHY GO, VEGAN?

To start with, let us say a Vegan diet consists of beans, grains, seeds, nuts, and of course, fruits, and vegetables. In fact, it is very similar to the Mediterranean diet, which has been touted for its health benefits, by using the same principles of consuming fruits, vegetables, and healthy fats.

The truth is that these fats are good fats. They are such as the ones found in nuts... yes, Nuts and foods such as avocados, boost High-density lipoprotein (HDL) cholesterol levels. This good cholesterol has been shown to help fight heart disease.

The main concern that often arises as an argument against a Vegan diet is that there will not be enough protein to maintain a healthy lifestyle. In fact, the average American people eat double as protein as is required of a healthy diet, and much of it is from red meat. However, receiving protein from grains and beans is healthier, and also minimizes risk for osteoporosis.

Anyway, recent studies have shown that 1 oz of almonds, or walnuts, contain just as much protein (6 g) as 1 oz of lean beef. Another point to consider is that the world's largest living land mammal, the Elephant, consumes an exclusively plant-based diet. If this enormous animal can not only survive, but thrive on a plant-based diet, it is proof enough that there is more than sufficient protein to be found inside a Vegan diet for a human being.

Further benefits of a Vegan diet, is that it has been viewed to prevent some number of diseases; these include Type 2 diabetes, High Blood Pressure, Breast cancer, Colon cancer, Rheumatoid Arthritis, and Macular Degeneration, to name a few. I have had personal results with eliminating High Blood Pressure by switching from a Vegetarian diet, to a Vegan diet.

By the way, you might be wondering what the difference is between a vegetarian diet and a vegan diet. Well, the major difference is that vegetarians may consume dairy products and eggs. But in veganism, on the other hand, there is no place for the consumption of any animal foods or its derivatives, including dairy and eggs. A vegan also avoids inedible animal-based produce, such as silk, wool, and leather. In other words, Vegetarianism is a diet, while veganism is a way of life (lifestyle).

Now, I have a confession to make... well not quite, but in support of the discuss here: having been on medication to regulate my blood pressure, I found that after embracing a Vegan diet, my blood pressure (bp.) dropped to normal levels on its own, and my need for medication was eliminated. Not surprising though, it took eight years later, for my doctor to agree that my choice of vegan diet paid off.

So How Do I Start the Transition Process?

Many people think this would be very difficult. That is ...eliminating all animal products cold turkey probably isn't for everyone. Well, I can say from experience, that there is nothing far from the truth than this! That being as it may, I need to emphasize the fact that you need to start small.

Hopefully, not many people are eating red meat anymore. I mean, after all the knowledge about their health hazards... Anyway, you can start by cutting out eggs for one week, and then progress to no dairy.

In fact, it has been observed that 75% of the world's population is lactose intolerant. Yes, many were unaware of this condition and their continuity of consuming dairy products can be linked to and responsible for many health issues, beginning with allergies.

There are also many Vegan versions of familiar foods that are available in your local grocery store. As Veganism has become more mainstream, there is soy and coconut based ice creams, Vegan cheese Vegan hot dogs Vegan mayonnaise (Veganaise is delicious), and also, a very wide variety of Vegan burgers.

Yes, what I am saying is that there is absolutely no reason to feel deprived in any way. In fact, one of the most amazing products to come out in recent years is called Gardein. A product of veganism!

Well, as you should have seen from the above, the benefits of a Vegan diet are disease prevention and even reversal in some case. Besides that, switching to a Vegan diet can also greatly minimize the toll on our planet's resources. The truth is that growing plants take far fewer resources than breeding animals for food.

Furthermore, by taking to veganism, you can assist in minimizing the toll on our whole environment. Factory Farming consumes enormous amounts of water, grain, petroleum, pesticides, and drugs. The grain used to feed cattle alone could be used to end the global world hunger problem.

In fact, going Vegan will also help you to look at an animal in the eye with a clear conscience. Go Vegan for the health benefits, for the planet, for the animals, but most of all, for yourself.

HOW THE KETOGENIC DIET WORKS

A lot of persons use a ketogenic diet for one reason or the other. It could be to shed weight or to treat epilepsy or Alzheimer's disease. Whatever the case may be, you will face the same thing when you take a keto diet.

Immediately you cut down on your consumption of carbs; you tend to notice that the amount of carbs in your food has reduced.

Before you cut the carb, the body usually burnt glucose, a product of the carbs. When you take in the carb, it is digested into glucose and used as an energy source. The glucose is transported by the blood around the body, especially the brain and the cells. The brain uses up glucose as an energy source to function well. Since you are eating a lot of foods that are high in carbs, the body continues to store up fats. Before you know it, you are increasing in weight and size.

When you have had enough and decided to lose weight, you can try out the keto diet and combine it with exercise, though not compulsory. A lot of persons use both to force their bodies into a state of ketosis quickly and burn off the burnt fat.

When you embrace keto, you toss away those foods that are high in carbs and embrace those that are high in fats.

Whatever you do while on a keto diet, your foods should be high in fats, moderate in protein, and low in carbs. Do not eat foods that are high in carbs because it could ruin your efforts. The body loves glucose, and immediately it sights high amount of carbs, even when it is in a state of ketosis, it throws the state of ketosis one side and embraces the glucose once more. When you eat foods that are high in protein, it is bad, as the body can transform excess protein to glucose.

What Happens When You Take Keto Friendly Diet

At first, when you consume a keto diet, you may notice keto flu. What is that? It is common to see a lot of those who are new to the ketogenic lifestyle feel some flu-like symptoms. Why does this happen?

When you take foods high in fats, and low in carbs, the body tries to adapt to the change. This means that the body won't have access to glucose any longer. The brain will try to adapt to its new energy source, ketones, and this can lead to headaches and nausea.

It could be as a result of you using the loo a lot. When a person is new to keto, he or she tends to urinate a lot. Why? It is simple. The person is losing a lot of electrolytes and water, hence needs replacement.

Once you start reducing the number of carbs you take, the body, especially the liver, takes the fats consumed and turn them to ketones and fatty acid. The ketones are the energy source, and they take the place of glucose. They are used by the body to carry out their daily activities. That's not all, as the body starts to use the stored-up fats. You see all those stored up fats that once remained untouched; the body starts to convert them to ketones. Before you know it, you are shedding weight effortlessly. At this stage, you are in ketosis. To prevent yourself from falling out of this state, you need to keep eating what you are eating.

KETO DIET BASICS FOR VEGAN

So now that we understand the concept of keto & veganism let's quickly dive into the brilliance of combining the two together. Both lifestyle choices are essentially designed to help us help our bodies perform in the best way possible. Both are also about clean eating; however, if you're applying the clean eating concepts of a keto diet to the ethical eating view of veganism can torpedo your health & wellness substantially.

A vegan can also opt to take up a ketogenic vegan diet. A vegan is an individual who prefers to eat plants such as potatoes, plant products, kale, & beans. Some vegans also don't eat or use honey. It is therefore evident that a vegan diet contains a high level of Carbs as a result of the sugar content & starch that is higher in plants than in animal products. As such, a ketogenic vegan diet may appear to be impossible. However, it can be done.

A ketogenic vegan diet has to be obtained from plant-based foods that are especially fatty, avoiding those that have high sugar or even starch contents. It is, however, a challenge, as the access to fatty plant-based foods commercially is less than plants that are either sugary or even starchy. This hinders food selection. Therefore, the sole difference between a ketogenic diet & a vegan ketogenic diet is the strict consumption of plants in the latter. The end goal, however, is the same.

The ketogenic diet lately has become the ultimate diet in terms of fat loss & ethical consumption, but meeting in the middle is never without compromise. The traditional keto diet is mainly based on consuming heavy animal fats. It would seem that the ketogenic diet & vegan diet are 2 opposite sides of a coin. This is because the ketogenic diet promotes the consumption of main fats & some protein, while maintaining very low levels of carbs, whereas a vegan diet is an ideology based on the premise that all living creatures, including animals, should be respected, & that the killing & consumption of animals & animal-based ingredients breaches this premise.

Depending on the side you're on, we are sure that you would have ample reason to support your cause. But the question is: could these diets actually overlap? Is it possible to follow the principles of veganism while enjoying the fat burning advantages of ketosis? The answer is YES! You can enjoy the best of both diets while still adhering to the ethical principles.

According to the conventional keto rules, a person is only allowed to consume 25G of net carbs every day. However, for a vegan following the ketogenic vegan diet, consuming about 30g of net carbs is easier to achieve, compared to the initial 20g especially when no animal products are involved, since all plant foods tend to have higher carbs as opposed to animal foods that are low in Carbs. So, consuming plant foods can even potentially increase the number of Carbs.

If you want to maintain the 15 to 20g carbs routine, it requires a strict diet plan or routine, especially on higher daily caloric intake. To maintain ketosis, it is always recommended to not go over 30g depending on your caloric needs, although there are a lot of vegan-keto people who consume up to 50g of Carbs& still lose weight while maintaining a healthy, cruelty-free lifestyle. It is also very dependent on the individual.

Below is the correct macronutrients ratio required for the keto diet

15 to 30 percent of calories should come from protein.

5 to 10 percent of calories should come from carbs.

60 to 75 percent of calories should come from fatty foods.

On a vegan diet, your main focus on consuming plant-based foods; however, not all plant-based foods are equal in nutritional value for your body, nor are they equal in energy value for your body.

When applying the ketogenic philosophy to your vegan diet, you can ensure that you're getting a stable level of green energy. The ketogenic lifestyle plan espouses the virtues of eating whole foods, which help keep you energized & full. Ketogenic-vegan foods ensure you're getting your nutrients without inundating your body with sugar.

We know that when you flood your body with sugar, you'll get a short sugar high, but then your energy levels will plummet. When your energy levels drop, you get hungry again quickly, & this could easily lead you to snack on quick snack foods that are high in fat & low on the nutrient scale. However, when you apply the ketogenic philosophy to the vegan diet, you'll ensure that you're only eating foods that are high in nutrients & energy without the influence of bad sugars.

HOW TO GET STARTED ON A HEALTHY KETOGENIC DIET

The ketogenic diet is a high fat, low carbohydrate diet with a moderate to a high amount of protein. It can be used to treat epilepsy. It is not an overnight fix. This is a difficult diet, and it can moderate electrical activity in the brain if used more than one to two years. This diet produces an effect similar to starvation and forces the body to burn fat instead of Carbs. Calories are strictly controlled so that weight is not lost or gained during the diet. Regular growth and repair of the body continue. This diet is heavily supplemented with vitamins and minerals. It should be done under the care of a registered dietician or physician. Fluids are restricted so that electrolytes do not get out of balance.

When glucose is not sufficient, the body burns fat. The fat is not completely burned, and ketones are formed. The high level of ketones formed seems to reduce or eliminate seizures in many people. People who are unable to control seizure activity can use this diet by other means. People can discontinue this diet after they have been seizure free for a period of approximately two years. This diet seems to alter the seizure threshold with the elevation of ketone levels. In 1998, Johns Hopkins Medical School released a study on the Ketogenic Diet. They showed the diet to significantly help eliminate the seizure activity in approximately one-third of the patients. Other patients showed reduced seizure activity.

In 2005, Emory University School of Medicine recently showed that this diet alters the genes involved in the energy metabolism of the brain. This action helps to stabilize neurons when seizure activity occurs. The diet increased the energy production in the hippocampus, helped the brain to become more resistant to reduced glucose levels, and increased the brain's ability to handle metabolism changes. This diet has the potential to treat Alzheimer's and Parkinson's Diseases.

Side effects of the Ketogenic Diet include dehydration, kidney stones, constipation, vomiting, increased cholesterol, lower growth rate, behavior changes, and mood changes. There are other diets to try if this diet is unsuccessful.

What You Need to Know Before Starting A Ketogenic Diet

There are some things everyone should know before they begin a ketogenic diet. They will help you to understand what you can expect and give you some guidance as you mentally prepare to do something your body is not accustomed to dealing with. Knowledge is power, and the more prepared you are before you begin, the more likely you will be to succeed at losing fat with the ketogenic diet.

Steps before getting started

Step One: Educate yourself on the ketogenic diet.

You have already taken the first step toward reaching your weight loss goal by reading this book. Congratulations! It is important to understand what you are getting in to and what to expect in order to meet your goals. While the ketogenic diet does have a high rate of success when it comes to people sticking to the diet, it does have its challenges to be prepared for. Once you get past the initial period of adjustment, things will get easier, but you don't want to go into it without some guidance first.

Step Two: Have a plan

Once you understand what the ketogenic diet is and how to do it, you need to have a plan, especially in the beginning. While your body is transitioning to using fat for fuel, there will be a lot of temptation to eat Carbs. We can get addictcd to wheat and sugar, so everyones' challenges are different. Some people will crave sugars while others could go without but crave bread. You will have to overcome those cravings whatever they may be.

A plan will get you through any weak moments you may face during the transition. It is always a good idea to try and keep planning things out in the future, but let's face it, life doesn't always allow us to plan every meal out in advance. Keep planning your meals and shopping ahead of time at least until you are no longer having cravings for Carbs.

Step Three: Get a water bottle and keep it with you

Your body will be changing the chemistry of how it functions, and this requires water to keep things moving well. Not only will your liver be working harder than it is used to in order to create ketones, but your brain needs to get that energy. If you are dehydrated, it makes things more difficult for your liver and can slow things down with getting the ketones to their destination.

In addition to helping your body function properly, you will need water to flush toxins out of your body. Many times the toxins that we encounter on a day to day basis accumulate in our fat stores, and when we start breaking fat cells down, we get an extra strong dose of these stored up toxins. It is vitally important to be well hydrated when this happens, so those toxins are removed from the body and not redeposit somewhere else or cause any harm. Many times when people are experiencing light-headedness and headaches during the initial phases of the ketogenic diet, it is a result of the toxins in their bloodstream, which need to be removed. To avoid this, you need to focus on drinking plenty of water. At a minimum, you should be drinking about two liters (or eight glasses) of water every day. Even if you aren't a water drinker, you need to start. Try just sipping on water throughout the day if you need to. You can also try tea or other zero calorie water add-ins if you can't stand plain water. You will appreciate not getting headaches from the diet as a result.

The bigger, the better when you get a water bottle. I recommend getting at least a 32-ounce bottle with a straw. It makes it much easier to get the water you need this way. If you have to refill your bottle frequently or open the lid every time you take a drink, it will reduce the amount of water you drink. If you have a water bottle handy that is big enough that you don't have keep refilling and a way to just sip on the water you will find yourself drinking it without even thinking about it pretty soon. I use a 40-ounce bottle with a straw and can easily drink four in a day. That's over four liters. You don't need to drink that much, but if you are doing it unconsciously, then your body needs that much water. Just keep in mind that the bottle has to be convenient enough for you to take with you everywhere you go. If a big 40-ounce bottle is too cumbersome, then get something smaller. It doesn't do you any good to have 40 ounces of water sitting at home because you didn't want to have to carry it everywhere.

Step four: Track all of your food in the beginning

When you first start the ketogenic diet, you probably won't have a very good idea of how many Carbs are in a lot of foods. You probably won't have a very good idea of how much protein or fat is anything either. Use a food tracker to count all of these nutrients so you get an idea of how much you are getting and you will start to learn what you can and can't have. There are plenty of food trackers out there, and some will even scan barcodes, so you don't have to look foods up. Once you start to learn how many carbs are in the foods that you normally eat, you can stop tracking everything. The ketogenic diet does not require you to limit calories because they will limit themselves. If you want more rapid weight loss and you want to limit calories, it would be a good idea to continue using a food tracker.

Step five: Get quality electrolytes

As previously mentioned, when your body goes into ketogenesis, your insulin will decrease, which lowers the amount of sodium your body will retain. Since you will be losing electrolytes, it is important to replace them. The best way to do this is with quality salts. Typical table salt has been purified so that it is pure sodium chloride. This helps to replenish the sodium that the body loses but does not replenish any other electrolytes that are lost in the process. Potassium and magnesium are also important electrolytes that must be replenished, so you don't get any of the negative side effects at the beginning of the ketogenic diet. Replacing pure table salt with Himalayan salt or Celtic salt can help replace some of those lost electrolytes since they contain magnesium and potassium in addition to sodium. It can also be helpful to drink zero calorie electrolyte drinks. Drinking bone broth is a more natural way of replacing electrolytes if you have the time to make it. Just make sure that you are getting plenty of electrolytes, however, you choose to do it, and you will feel fewer symptoms while adjusting to the ketogenic diet.

Step six: Avoid artificial sweeteners

It is a good idea, in the beginning, to plan on avoiding foods with artificial sweeteners in them. This is to help you get over the sugar addiction that you likely have. Even though you may not be eating actual sugar, the sweetness will remind your brain that it is craving sugar and make things harder for you during the transition. This is more of a recommendation than a requirement. Some people have a strong sugar addiction and will struggle if they get artificial sweeteners while others won't be affected at all. Plan for success though and just try to avoid them while your body is getting used to the changes.

HEALTH BENEFITS OF KETO VEGAN DIET

The number of vegans goes up every year, and not only because people are concerned about animal exploitation. There are a number of health reasons to make the switch and cut out meat, dairy, and other animal products:

Improved Digestion:

Vegan staples like vegetables and fruit are full of fiber, which is essential for a healthy digestive system. On the other hand, animal-based foods, especially dairy, are known to cause chronic gut problems like constipation and inflammation. When you cut those out of your diet and start eating a lot more vegetables, your digestion will improve significantly. If you didn't eat a lot of fiber before, take it slow. When your body isn't used to a high volume of fiber, it can cause issues like diarrhea. Even chewing really thoroughly can help prevent some of the initial symptoms.

Healthier Skin:

In addition to fiber, fruit and vegetables are packed with water, which will keep you hydrated. That shows on your skin, which can begin glowing and healing from inflammation very soon after you switch to a vegan diet. Plant-based foods are high in other vitamins and nutrients that your skin loves, like vitamin A and vitamin E. the best foods for skin include beets, avocados, dark leafy greens, oranges, and apples.

More Energy:

If you struggle with fatigue, a vegan diet can boost your energy. This is most likely because of your healthier digestion system. When it's working harder to digest meat and dairy, it uses up a lot of your energy store, so all you feel like doing is taking a nap. Plant-based foods are much lighter, digest quicker, and contain energy-boosting nutrients like iron, potassium, calcium, and vitamin E and K. dark leafy greens are very effective at raising your energy levels.

Protection against Genetic Diseases:

Certain diseases are most likely linked to genetics, like

type 2 diabetes. However, some studies show that a plant-based diet might help combat your genes and prevent disease from developing. This is because of various compounds and antioxidants in plants that fight against free radical cells, which cause cell damage, inflammation, and trigger illnesses.

Protection against Cancer:
Studies show that vegans have lower cancer rates than meat-eaters or even vegetarians. In 2014, a study funded by the National Cancer Institute found that vegan women had a 34% lower chance of getting cervical, breast, or ovarian cancer. Another study indicated that people who eat are at a higher risk of colon and prostate cancers. Cutting out meat and dairy while embracing significantly more vegetables, fruit, and other plant-based foods could provide protection from a variety of cancers.

The vegan diet, which cuts out all animal products, has benefits such as improved energy, protection against diseases, Protection against Cancer, healthier skin, and improved digestion.

KETO SIDE EFFECTS

At this point, you might be wondering what kind of toll such a significant change to your diet is going to take on how you feel, especially if you are used to consuming higher amounts of carbohydrates. Your body may have built up a stock of carbohydrate-active enzymes, and therefore might not be well-equipped to break down and store large volumes of fat, or to deal with a sudden shortage of glucose. As a result, your body has to produce an entirely new supply of enzymes. After an adjustment period, your body will naturally begin to use your reserves of glucose, stored in the liver and muscles, for energy. This can lead to lethargy and sluggishness.

Many people cite dizziness, headaches, and irritability as early side effects of the keto diet, particularly during the first seven days. This is due to the depletion of electrolytes from your system, which is, of course, another reason to drink plenty of fluids and replenish your sodium levels. Since sodium helps retain water in the body, many dieticians recommend upping your salt intake significantly.

The keto flu: We've already mentioned the keto flu, but as it is one of the most common side effects of the keto diet, let's examine it in a little more detail. Despite the name, the keto flu (also known as the 'low-carb flu') is not a kind of influenza. It is so-called because many newcomers to the keto diet experience a number of flu-like symptoms in the early stages of their keto transformation.

There are two main reasons why keto flu occurs:

1. More frequent trips to the bathroom: Increased urination leads to a considerable loss of electrolytes and water. You can preemptively combat this problem by drinking a bouillon cube dissolved in water.

2. Withdrawal: Remember, your body is going through a major transition! It now has to adjust to a significant drop in carb intake and create new enzymes to process increased amounts of fat. This is hard work for your

body, and you may feel lethargic as a result. To ease this, you should try decreasing your carb intake gradually, rather than quitting cold turkey.

Increasing your water consumption and replacing lost electrolytes will effectively combat or even eradicate the keto flu. At the beginning of your transition, you should try to eat less than 15 grams of carbohydrates a day, then decrease this number little by little over time. Nothing worth doing is easy, but thankfully, the drawbacks of the keto diet are few and, for the most part, easily alleviated. The same cannot be said for many other fad diets out there!

Here are some other notable side effects of the ketogenic diet, and suggestions as to how you can deal with them.

Fatigue and irritability – High ketone levels can positively impact your physical wellbeing in a number of ways, but they are also linked to increased tiredness and quicker exertion during exercise. Make sure you are getting enough sleep during the early days of your transition and avoid particularly strenuous exercise if necessary.

'Brain fog' – Your altered metabolism and hormonal state may cause decreased mental clarity or 'brain fog.' This is a common side effect of total carbohydrate withdrawal, which is why you should avoid going cold turkey and instead decrease your carbohydrate intake gradually and steadily.

Change in lipids – An important tenet of the ketogenic diet is not only to up your fat intake but also to watch what kinds of fats you are consuming. Saturated fats are known to increase cholesterol levels, so make sure they do not outbalance the non-saturated fats in your diet.

Micronutrient deficiencies – Low-carb foods are often lacking in important nutrients like magnesium, potassium, and iron. Taking supplements is an excellent way of compensating for this.

Ketoacidosis – If your diet is poorly-planned, you may

be at risk of developing ketoacidosis, which is characterized by extremely high ketone levels. This is especially harmful to people living with diabetes, so make sure you organize your diet to keep your ketone levels within a healthy range. Additionally, it is important to know how to recognize the signs. These include shortness of breath, pain in the abdomen, confusion, nausea, vomiting, and weakness if you experience any combination of these symptoms while on the ketogenic diet, seek medical attention immediately.

Muscle loss – Decreased carbohydrate consumption means your body may draw on protein in your muscles for energy, leading to a decrease in muscle mass. In particular, this side effect is associated with those who engage in rigorous workouts, so consider scaling back your exercise routine if muscle loss is a major concern for you.

WHAT TO EAT ON A VEGAN KETO DIET

As a vegan entering into the Keto diet, you'll want to pay special attention to your balance of food groups in order to get the proper nutrition out of a Keto vegan diet. Your vitamins and supplements will definitely help boost your energy levels and keep your nutrition on track, but especially when it comes to fats, you need to make sure a vegan eating Keto that you know where your best options are for plant-based fats. The more fats you can eat during Keto, the better—you'll feel much more full, and help yourself reach Ketosis as quickly as possible to start burning fat. The best plant-based sources of healthy, whole fats are actually oils. From olive oil to coconut oil, whole fats in the oil are one of the best ways to add to your meals on the vegan Keto diet without busting your calorie count. While coconut oil is the lowest in terms of calories, it has a lower smoke point than olive oil, so be careful when you're cooking to choose the right one. Both avocado meat and avocado oil have plenty of healthy fats, and they're a great example of how you can remember to eat your fatty foods—most of these oils are extracted from a healthy source, and the source foods are good for you too! Flaxseed oil and flaxseeds will boost your healthy fat content, and sesame seeds are just as delicious as sesame oil. Eating plenty of nuts and seeds alongside cooking with healthy oils will really make an impact on your journey towards Ketosis and your energy levels if you encounter the Keto flu. Fats are going to make up about eighty percent of your vegan Keto diet, so take note of all the possible ways you can get them. Proteins are next, and while you might be thinking, you know which vegetables you're going to go for exactly—be careful. The Keto diet limits certain things like black beans and chickpeas that are staples in vegan cuisine. Instead, you're going to need to get creative with your vegetables and with the...soy products? That's right. If you're a tofu-munching, tempeh-loving vegan, the Keto diet is about to become your new favorite style of eating. Soy products are packed with natural proteins—there are two grams of protein per ounce of tofu. Soy products are also incredibly easy to make tasty and delicious since they tend to soak up whatever they're cooked in (like healthy, fatty oil!). If tofu isn't for you, there are plenty of high protein vegetables that will help you conquer Keto veganism. Kale, spinach, and asparagus are packed with protein, and three great examples of how you can once again use color to determine which of your foods are best. Dark green vegetables are your healthiest, with lighter green veggies coming next. Bok choy, zucchini, green onions, Brussel sprouts, edamame, and snap peas are great ingredients to keep in mind - but don't forget about your light green lettuces! Cabbage is one of the healthiest foods in the world and makes a fantastic addition to many vegan Keto recipes. Cucumber, eggplants, and olives aren't just the delicious staples of the Mediterranean diet. Your vegan Keto experience will be so much better with a Keto Eggplant Vegan-Parmesan. Cauliflower can replace just about anything, and it should—per one ounce, you get a whopping half a gram of protein. Even stranger than cauliflower is the high protein content of the almost translucent watercress: in just one hundred g, watercress gives you two point three grams of protein. After lighter greens and whites, all your orange, yellow, and red vegetables tend to be very high in Carbs (with the exception of tomatoes). And if it grows in the ground—leave it there. Legumes and root veggies have too much sugar.

WHAT NOT TO EAT ON A VEGAN KETO DIET

While you'll obviously be avoiding any animal products while you're eating a strictly vegan Keto diet, there are a few key changes you'll want to make in order to avoid sabotaging your own weight loss goals. While it's important to avoid certain foods as a vegan, it's even more important to avoid certain foods as a vegan eating a Keto diet, because if you aren't careful, you'll fail to reach Ketosis and won't begin to burn fat rapidly. The Keto diet itself limits a few foods right out of the gate, and they are all foods you'll likely recognize: processed foods, alcohol, added sugars, sodas, and artificial sweeteners. But there are some foods you're more likely used to seeing on recommended lists—the Keto diet limits all fruits, although a few occasional servings of specific types are allowed. Grains and heavy starches are also limited, as well as starchy vegetables like potatoes and sweet potatoes. If you're starting to understand why the Keto vegan diet is such a commitment, that's a good thing. The more you know about what you're getting into, the more likely it is that you'll be successful on the other side. The vegan Keto diet also urges you to limit your intake of legumes like black beans and chickpeas, as well as all diet foods that are low in fat content, but high in sugar content. Even the natural sweetener agave gets kicked to the curb, with too much glucose content. Leave your condiments behind as well—most salad dressings, sauces, and bottled condiments are packed full of artificial sugar. Speaking of salad dressings and condiments, if you didn't already know, these are two of the most popular foods that companies like to hide animal derivatives inside. Animal derivatives could be anything from bones used in gelatin (yes, that's true) or food coloring made out of the bodies of insects. Keep an eye on your salad dressing labels for anchovies, sardines, eggs, bacon fat, "cochineal" coloring in any red dyes beginning with a capital "E," and fish oils. Watch out for barbecue sauces too—they like to add beef bouillon and other animal products to "beef" up the taste.

IS IT RIGHT FOR YOU?

While the keto diet is a great and effective tool for weight loss, it may not be the right diet for you. Chances are, before reading this book, you had heard about the keto diet and decided that it was just another fad that won't last, but it has been followed for over 100 years. You are already aware of all the health benefits that the diet brings, and all of this is due to ketosis. But it is this ketone adaptation that can cause some safety problems that you need to keep in mind. This is why I have provided you with this chapter because it may not be a good idea for everybody. The following are some situations where a ketogenic diet may be dangerous. While you may still be able to follow it, you will want to exercise caution and do so under a doctor's supervision.

Pregnant or Nursing

There aren't a lot of studies done on the effects of a keto diet on a pregnant woman. Some studies, though, have found that some side effects could include weight loss, anemia, nutrient deficiency, hormonal changes, dehydration, inadequate growth in the fetus, and constipation.

Prolong ketosis while pregnant could end up causing developmental problems for the baby that can end up affecting the development of their brain and increases the risk of defects, such as spina bifida. Due to the problems that it could cause the baby, doctors do not recommend this diet for pregnant women.

Much like with a pregnant woman, there aren't too many studies about what keto can do to a nursing woman. Most women who are nursing or pregnant often need more protein and fiber than other women. The increased fiber helps to support the development and growth of the fetus, helps with their digestion, and provides both mom and baby with the vitamins and minerals they need.

Since we don't know for certain the exact results of a ketogenic diet on nursing women, it is best to follow a moderate carb intake that is safe for the mother and the baby.

Medication-Caused Hypoglycemia
The most common hypoglycemia-causing medications are:

1. Insulin

2. Sulphonylureas, such as glibenclamide, tolbutamide, gliclazide, glipizide, and glimepiride.

3. Glinides, such as nateglinide or repaglinide.

4. All of these medications are made to help increase insulin in the body. This will then lower a person's blood sugar levels if you are following a ketogenic diet while on these medications, it could increase your odds of developing hypoglycemia. It is important that you speak to your doctor so that both of you can work together to prevent you from developing hypoglycemia before you start keto.

Making sure that you take regular blood glucose tests will give you the ability to spot and avoid developing hypoglycemia. You will have to perform tests more often than normal while your body works to adjust to the change of carbohydrate intake.

Diabetes or Blood Sugar Problems

There are plenty of people who suffer from diabetes or blood sugar problems that can follow a keto diet without any problems. There are some, however, who try to follow a keto diet and will suffer from low blood sugar when they first start. This can turn out to be dangerous if you are unable to stabilize your blood sugar while on diabetes medications.

There is a lot of evidence that shows that diabetes can be slowed or prevents through a healthy diet and exercise. To be on the safe side, people who have a history of hypoglycemia, prediabetes, or diabetes should consult with their doctor before they begin a ketogenic diet.

Changes in your diet and weight loss could mean that you need to change your diabetes medication dosage. Only your doctor can make these. You should never change your medication without talking with your doctor first.

Other Medications

The majority of medications won't cause significant risk, but you should still to do some research and speak with your doctor to make sure there won't be any problems. Your doctor will know if they need to change the dosage. Blood pressure medications could end up needing to be regulated more by your physician because a keto diet could cause your blood pressure to drop too low.

Underweight or Nutrient Deficient

The ketogenic diet is meant as a way to lose weight, and weight loss tends to happen quickly. If you are currently underweight, have vitamin or mineral deficiencies due to not eating right, or have suffered from past eating disorders, this is not the right diet for you. If your BMI is in the underweight range and you want to follow a keto diet to improve your blood sugar levels, and you don't want to lose weight, please talk to your doctor to help you to modify the diet to ensure that your weight isn't affected.

If you tend to lose weight easily, a diet with more complex carbs along with plenty of healthy fats and proteins is the best thing. If you have ever undergone gastric bypass surgery, the ketogenic diet may be dangerous because of the risk of nutrient deficiencies that can happen from not consuming enough calories.

Children

While there have been many children suffering from epileptic seizures who have been treated with a ketogenic diet, they were under medical supervision. There are many different things that you need to remember before starting a ketogenic diet for a child is to make sure that the macronutrients are balanced and appropriate for them. You absolutely must speak with a doctor or dietitian before you allow your child to start a keto diet.

Kidney Disease or Stones

The keto diet has the ability to cause kidney stones. If you already have a history of kidney disease, it probably isn't worth it to try and follow a ketogenic diet. If you have a history of any type of kidney disease, you have to talk with your doctor before you start this type of diet. Your doctor will need to keep an eye on your creatinine/calcium ratio to make sure that you aren't suffering from complications like nephrolithiasis, which is very dangerous calcium levels in your kidneys.

Gallstones or Gall Bladder Removal

People who suffer from gallstones are often told to stay away from fat, but that isn't necessarily the case anymore. The NHS says that a low-fat diet can cause gallstone growth. If you already suffer from gallstones, consuming more fat could cause more pain. If you are interested in a ketogenic diet, you may want to slowly start the diet or wait until your gallstones have been removed.

A study in 2014 found that high-fat diets could prevent the formation of gallstones, which could be another long-term benefit of this diet. The gall bladder has bile in it that will help your body to break down fats, so it may not seem like a smart idea to follow a high-fat diet like a ketogenic diet. There are plenty of people, though, that have had their gall bladder removed that have successfully followed the diet without any adverse effects.

Enzyme Deficiency or Defect

These are both very rare problems, but there are two big contraindications of the ketogenic diet called pyruvate carboxylase and porphyria deficiency. These are both caused by issues with the production of lipid and heme metabolism. Heme is part of the hemoglobin that carries oxygen out of the lungs and into other areas of your body.

People who suffer from these disorders will also suffer from deficiencies with some enzymes that make it hard for them to metabolize large amounts of fatty acids. They are then transported to the cell's mitochondria to make energy. If you follow this type of diet and suffer from these deficiencies or other types of beta oxidations defects, it can create dangerous complications like irregular heartbeats, nervous system deterioration, and mental changes.

Free fatty acids will build up, but the body won't be able to sue them for energy, and this is why it becomes dangerous. People who have pyruvate carboxylase and porphyria deficiency need a good supply of glucose to provide their organs with energy. If there is no glucose present because of this diet, some life-threatening problems can occur. This is known as a catabolic crisis. To avoid these problems, if you have a family history of mitochondrial disorders or you think you may have these conditions, you need to have a doctor test you before even thinking about starting a ketogenic diet.

KETOGENIC DIET TIPS

Following the Ketogenic Diet is as easy as counting to three. As long as you have good self-discipline and self-control, you can successfully abide by the Ketogenic Diet. Read the following to know the tips and tricks of following this diet.

How easy is it to follow the Ketogenic Diet?
There is really no profound secret to following a diet except to have self-discipline, self-control, and a vision. These three main traits are what will keep you on the right track towards achieving your goals – whether to lose weight, burn fat, or maintain a healthy lifestyle. However, it is also true that humans lose track of their goals once in a while because life happens.

Either you focus on your job and you don't have time to fix your meals or you start your own family and your own goals take a back seat. All of these happen and all constitute and contribute to the failure of keeping track of one's diet. Taking into consideration the happenings of daily life, here are some tips that will keep you on track with regard to following your Ketogenic Diet:

1. Be Patient - It takes time to lose weight:
Patience is the key to staying loyal to your Ketogenic Diet. The results of your diet plan cannot be achieved or be seen overnight. It takes time to lose weight, especially since this diet plan is not a crash-type of diet. Give it a month or so before you see some changes in your body frame, weight, and disposition.

One way to achieve patience is by being honest and true to yourself. Think of it this way - You didn't attain your current weight overnight, right? So, what makes you think that you can lose it overnight? Gaining may come easy for a lot of people, but losing weight takes longer. Keep that in mind. Give it some time.

2. Get Enough Sleep:
If you think diet alone is enough to help you shed pounds and build muscle, then you're wrong. Getting enough hours of sleep is crucial to help you achieve

the body that you want to achieve. Diet and sleep are two activities that need to be practiced to lose weight. A lot of internal changes in the body happen during sleep, so even if you follow your Ketogenic Diet to the key but do not get at least 7 hours of sleep every night (yes at night!), then your hard work will go to waste.

3. Clean Your Kitchen Cupboards:
Once you decide to follow the Ketogenic Diet, you must also commit yourself to clean and free your kitchen of foods that will tempt you off your path to a healthier life. Remove items that are high in carbohydrates as well as items with empty calories. Yes, the Ketogenic Diet may have a high-fat content, but these are not coming from the saturated fat present in junk food. You also need to remove items high in sugar and high in sodium.

4. Hydrate Well - drink lots of water:
You need to drinks lots of water to aid in cleansing your body. Your diet in itself is cleansing your body of excess toxins, but to wash these toxins out of your body, you need to drink water. Take in at least three

liters of water a day to keep your excretory system active.

5. Look for a Partner:
There is no other better way to stay loyal to a diet than committing to it with a partner. It is even better if your diet partner is someone who lives with you like a spouse, sibling, or best friend. This way, you can check each other's meal plans, help each other during difficult days, and encourage each other to stick with the diet plan.

6. Weigh Yourself Every Other Week:
You decided to follow the Ketogenic Diet. Yes, you want to see results as soon as you can, but please do not obsess overseeing the results a few days after your first day in. You can weigh yourself but do this every other week only. It is more encouraging for you to schedule a day and time every other week for your weighing duties. Weighing every other week gives you a more favorable result than checking every day.

DIFFICULTIES THAT ARISE DURING THE DIET

So, at this point, you've probably already begun your keto vegan journey. And by now you've most likely run into some of the obstacles that make the entire thing almost tedious. It's normal to encounter difficulties along the way; nothing good tends to come easy.

You might find it difficult starting the vegan keto diet, especially since your body needs to adjust to the new normal (at least for the period you'll spend on the diet).

Most times, the problems you might be facing could be easily solved by increasing your water and salt intake; although not every challenge is as easy as that. And when you do this, you'll find that your problems might reduce considerably.

Here are some notable side effects of the diet and their possible solution;

Induction (Keto) Flu

When most individuals start the high-fat low-carb diet, one of the first issues they experience is the keto flu (as it's popularly called). It occurs within the first week – around day 2-4.

The term flu comes from the fact that the ailment mimics flu-like symptoms. During this transition period, it's normal to feel tired, lethargic, headaches, nausea, and lack of motivation or 'brain fog.' Some people even feel irritated by anyone in their immediate vicinity.

The good about these symptoms is that they don't usually last for long and disappear on their own after a few days. It's also possible to avoid them altogether by staying hydrated and consuming more sodium. You could easily add a half teaspoon of salt to a large cup of water and drink it. Repeating this practice would help you feel less miserable when you start experiencing these symptoms.

Leg Cramps

This side effect isn't uncommon for individuals beginning any strict low-carb diet. The issue might seem minor at first, but it can be painful to deal with for some. Leg cramps occur as a result of the loss of minerals (especially magnesium) through increased urination.

The best way to handle the situation is by drinking lots of fluid and salt; if needed, get magnesium supplements for the time being. But if neither options work, you might want to consider increasing your carb consumption by a little bit; although this might affect your diet.

Constipation

Having difficulty stooling is another effect of the low-carb diet – especially during the first week. Your digestive system is taking the time to adapt to its new situation, and as a result, it becomes increasingly difficult to get rid of wastes.

As usual, you are drinking lots of water and salt tends

to ease the problem. Also, you need to get a good source of quality fiber to consume since most of the previous options involved high-carbs. Eat plenty of non-starchy vegetables or dissolve psyllium seed husks to a glass of water and drink it.

Bad Breath

While on the keto vegan diet, there's a high chance that your breath would start smelling different. The almost fruity smell comes from acetone – a ketone body, and it's a sure sign that your body is already burning tons of fats and converting them to ketones as fuel.

However, not everyone on the keto diet experiences the lousy breath effect. For some people, it manifests in their sweat, especially when they work out too much. The good news here is that this side effect doesn't last long (a week or two). Once the body adapts to the fat, it stops leaking ketones through the sweat and breath.

On the off-chance that the bad breath doesn't go away

(yes, it's been known to happen once in a while), here are several ways to remedy the issue.

i. Drink lots of fluids

ii. Practice good oral hygiene (brush maybe thrice a day)

iii. Get a breath-freshener to mask the smell

iv. Wait and see if it's temporary (most times it is)

v. Slightly reduce the degree of your ketosis by eating a bit more carbs (it shouldn't stop your progress though)

Increased Heart Rate

It's not surprising to experience heart palpitations during the first couple of weeks on the low-carb diet. It shows your heart is beating harder – which isn't abnormal. It means there's a reduction of circulating fluid in the bloodstream and your heart is working harder to pump more blood to maintain the pressure.

As usual, drinking more fluids help ease this

symptom. The increased heart pumping could also be because of the new changes to the body and the stress it has to endure. But, if you already have previous cardiac issues, you might need to consult your physician for more information on the situation.

Reduction in Physical Performance

During the initial weeks of starting the keto vegan diet, your physical performance might be severely reduced mostly due to fat-adaptation and lack of fluids and salts.

The fat-adaptation process might take a little time for the body to adjust, but it can be improved by exercising more during the diet. The benefits of the low-carb, high-fat diet can be seen most times in long-distance races and other sports that require pushing your endurance levels.

This happens because the body's fat stores are a lot greater than the glycogen ones. It shows once the body becomes fat-adapted, athletes could perform for more extended periods without the need for external energy. As they exercise, their body uses up the fat as fuel.

It frees them from having to activate their gastrointestinal organs during the activity, and a large portion of blood flow would be directed to the muscles. Plus, a low-carb diet comes with a reduction of body fats which allows the athletes to feel lighter; increasing their output.

Temporary Loss of Hair

This symptom could occur in pretty much any major diet change, and it happens for different reasons, none of which is permanent. It's common in low-carb diets because of the restriction of calories.

Fortunately, the hair loss doesn't happen to everyone and is barely noticeable with people that experience it. Naturally, individuals already experience little amounts of hair loss when new hair follicles push the old ones out – but we don't notice it since it's infinitesimal.

When the body starts going through stress, more

strands are lost than usual due to numerous reasons all having to do with the diet. There's really not much to do about this symptom than eating nutritious veggies and sleeping well since the effects are temporary. Also, try to reduce other external sources of stress to the body.

Elevated Cholesterol

The great news about the keto vegan diet is that it leads to an improved cholesterol profile, resulting in a lower risk of cardiac diseases. One of the positive effects is that it elevates HDL reduces signs of atherosclerosis.

Even though it's rare, very few people (partly due to genetics) still end up with high elevations of LDL and total cholesterol; none of which could be considered normal. This potential risk can be taken care of through little steps like;

- Avoid drinking bulletproof coffee:
- This brand of beverage involves adding MCT oil, butter, or coconut fat to coffee. Don't

consume significant amounts of fatty drinks when you're not hungry. It'll play a vital role in normalizing your cholesterol levels

- Use more unsaturated fats (avocados, olive oil)
- It'll go a long way in lowering your already high cholesterol.
- Eat only when you're hungry
- Intermittently fasting once in a while should help in reducing your levels
- And if nothing else works for you, consider looking for a less strict diet.

Low-Carb and Alcohol Intolerance

Most people on low-carb diets tend to lose their tolerance for alcohol and get intoxicated quickly. That's why you need to be careful when drinking alcohol on a low-carb diet. You could always think of it as a way of saving money at the bar since you only need half as many drinks to get a buzz going.

There's no apparent cut reason yet for this phenomenon. It could be that the liver is too busy producing ketones to have the time or capacity to burn the alcohol you're consuming.

Or it could be that sugar (fructose) and alcohol are almost similarly broken down in the liver, and consuming a reduced quantity could make the liver briefly less adapted to breaking down the alcohol.

Regardless of what the science behind the process is, the fact is that keto diet reduces your tolerance for alcohol. So, always remember to be careful if you decide to drink.

Period Changes

While on the keto diet, some women might notice a change in their menstrual cycle. In some cases, it becomes irregular, while in some others it stops altogether. This situation occurs mostly due to rapid weight loss due to drops in gonadotropin-releasing hormone (GRH), estrogen, progesterone, luteinizing hormone (LH), and follicle-stimulating hormone

(FSH).

When this disruption to the menstrual period occurs, serious side effects tend to follow, such as; low bone density, depression, anxiety, and sexual dysfunction. If your period suddenly becomes irregular or stops entirely during this diet, you need to consult your doctor as soon as possible because it's a bad sign.

However, there's a plus side to this for women with polycystic ovary syndrome (PCOS). It's a loophole of sorts. The keto diet helps people suffering from PCOS in regulating their periods.

Whether you have any preexisting health issues, it's best to ask your physician if it's okay for you to embark on the keto vegan diet since they're so many things to consider. If you suffer from any type of kidney dysfunction, Type-1 or 2 Diabetes, or a heart defect, you might want to avoid the diet or get approval from your doctor first.

Ketosis is actually beneficial to individuals suffering from hyperglycemia issues; although they have to be careful of their blood sugar and check their glucose levels multiple times daily.

Reasons Why You Might not be Losing Weight on the Keto Vegan Diet

There are so many possible reasons why you're not shedding pounds even

after spending weeks doing the keto diet, and you're following the guidelines. Before you decide to give up and go back to your carbs and bread, consider these following explanations.

1) You probably never entered ketosis

This idea might seem crazy to you, especially when you've spent all these while slashing your carb levels and curbing your sweet tooth. But if you can't see any visible results after spending so long on a diet, then you need to make sure that you're doing the right thing. So, hit the pause button and test your urine or blood to see if there's ketone in your bloodstream. And if it turns out that you're not in ketosis, try increasing your daily fat content from 75% to around

90% for better results.

2) You're consuming more proteins than necessary
The keto vegan diet is high-fat and not high-protein; try not to mistake the two things. As a result, you need a moderate amount of proteins and more fatty foods. Consuming high amounts of proteinic food could prevent you from achieving ketosis – or even kick you out of it if you're already there.

3) You're probably missing hidden carb sources
Vegetables and nuts are keto-friendly, and all, but some of them contain high amounts of carbs. If you don't pay enough attention to the contents of most of the food you eat, you will end up surpassing your daily carb content. You need to limit your daily carbohydrate calories to 2-5%, which means you need to keep track of almost every single bite. No one said this diet would be easy.

4) High daily calorie intake
Regardless of which nutrient group you're getting your calories from, once it's higher than what your

body needs at a particular time, the rest is stored as fat. And that means you'll gain weight even if you're in ketosis.

If you want your diet to become successful, you need to pay close attention to everything you eat and do. It's crucial because one misstep could affect your entire result.

Debunking Some Common Keto Vegan Myths

Despite the apparent benefits of the diet, there's still some air of uncertainty around it. Some people don't feel assured of the merits of following a high-fat, low-carb meal plan, especially when it combines veganism to the mix. They think it limits their already slim food-pool.

Let's take a look at the top four myths;

#1: Eating lots of Fatty Foods makes you Fat

This common misconception is probably popular due to years of marketing of low-fat products to consumers. Most health ads and commercial feature greasy burgers and grease as a way of deterring people from consuming foods containing high fats.

When in actuality, the problem originates from meals laden with high amounts of Carbs and processed sugar. They cause most of the health complications that are linked with diabetes and other diseases.

As soon as you kick your unhealthy habits and stick to a quality high-fat diet that includes avocados, nuts, and vegetables, your body will stop storing excessive amounts of glucose used as body fat. And unlike with a high-carb diet, eating healthy fatty foods keep you satisfied and curb your cravings. Once your appetite is suppressed, you'll be less likely to consume many calories.

#2: The diet won't be sustained since it's deficient in some vitamins and minerals

If you follow the keto vegan diet correctly, it contains all the essential micronutrients your body needs to function correctly. Some people might wonder how possible it is to skip some fruits (oranges and apples) and still remain healthy.

It's easy since there are several low-carb vegetables (spinach, arugula, and berries) that offer all the essential vitamins and minerals you get from those particular fruits; minus the sugar.

#3: As long as you keep your carb levels low, you can eat as much protein

As we mentioned earlier, consuming so many proteins is a common rookie misstep during the keto vegan diet. Excess amount of proteins in the body leads to gluconeogenesis, which causes it to convert the surplus amino acids to glucose. And this act prevents ketosis from happening. On the ketogenic diet, fat is the body's primary source of fuel. Remember that there's no such thing as 'essential carbs,' only 'essential fats.'

#4: The ketogenic diet causes electrolyte deficiency and dehydration

While this myth has a little bit of truth to it, there are still ways to avoid it from happening in the first place.

The deficiency of electrolytes in the body is a pretty valid concern and can be remedied by drinking lots of water, salt, and taking supplements.

As long as you follow all the rules governing the keto vegan diet, you shouldn't encounter many difficulties achieving ketosis successfully. The process is long and sometimes challenging, but in the end, the results are worth the entire ordeal.

BREAKFAST

01. Astonishing Vegan Hemp Seed Yogurt

Servings:8

Preparation Time: 200 minutes

Cooking Time: 0 minutes

Ingredients

- ¾ cup of hulled hemp seeds
- 3 cups of boiling water
- ¼ cup of lemon juice
- 2 teaspoon of xanthan gum
- Stevia as needed

Directions:

1. Take a pan and bring water to a boil
2. Take 1 cup of boiling water and mix them with hemp seeds in a blender
3. Process until the smooth lump-free mixture

forms

4. While the blender is still processing, add xanthan gum and 2 cups of the remaining water

5. Process for 30 seconds more

6. Add lemon juice and blend for a little longer

7. Pour into a container and allow it to chill for 2-3 hours

8. Once the yogurt has set,

enjoy!

Nutrition Values:

Calories: 166

Fat: 12G

Carbs: 4g

Protein: 10g

02. Sensual Portobello Mushrooms

Preparation Time: 10 minutes

Cooking Time: 10 minutes

Servings:2

Ingredients:

- 2 Portobello mushrooms
- ½ cup of extra virgin olive oil
- 2 tablespoons of chopped onion
- 3 minced clove of garlic
- 3 tablespoons of balsamic vinegar

Directions:

1. Carefully clear up mushrooms and remove stems
2. Keep the mushrooms for later use
3. Place the caps on a plate (gills upward)
4. Take a small sized bowl and add onion,

vinegar, oil, and garlic

5. Mix everything well
6. Pour the mixture over the mushrooms caps and allow it to stand for about 60 minutes
7. Grill for about 10 minutes over your grill
8. Enjoy the grilled Portobello Mushrooms!

Nutrition Values:

Calories: 177

Fat: 14

Carbs: 7

Protein: 2.4g

03. Surprisingly Keto Tomato Tart

Servings:8

Preparation Time: 10 minutes

Cooking Time: 25 minutes

Ingredients

For Crust

- ½ a cup of coconut oil
- ¾ cup of coconut flour
- ½ a teaspoon of salt
- the mixture of 1 tablespoon of ground flaxseed + ¼ cup of water

For Filling

- 4 ounce of heirloom tomatoes
- 3 ounce of vegan cheese substitute
- Black pepper and other herbs as needed

Directions:

1. Pre-heat your oven to 350 degrees Fahrenheit
2. Take a 9-inches pan and add all of the crust ingredients
3. Spread them out evenly and bake for 15-20 minutes until the crust starts to set

4. Remove the crust
5. Spread the vegan cheese shredded over the crust
6. Slice up tomatoes into ¼ inch slices and arrange them on top of the Cheese
7. Sprinkle cracked pepper, oregano, basil and any other herbs of your choice
8. Cover and bake for 20-25 minutes until the cheese has melted, and the tomatoes are tender
9. Allow it to cool and enjoy!

Nutrition Values:

Calories: 212

Fat: 18G

Carbs: 5g

Protein: 2G

04. Kalamata Olive Tapenade

Preparation Time: 15 minutes

Cooking Time: 0 minute

Servings:4

Ingredients:

- 3 peeled garlic cloves
- 1 cup of pitted kalamata olives
- 2 tablespoons of capers
- 3 tablespoons of chopped fresh parsley
- 2 tablespoons of lemon juice
- 2 tablespoons of extra virgin olive oil
- Salt as needed
- Pepper as needed

Directions:

1. Take a food processor and add garlic cloves
2. Pulse them well until they are fully minced
3. Add olives, olive oil, capers, parsley, lemon

juice to the food processor and blend them well until the whole mixture is finely chopped up

4. Season with some pepper and salt
5. Serve and enjoy!

Nutrition Values:

Calories: 81

Fat: 8g

Carbs: 3g

Protein: 0.5g

05. Silly Scallion Pancakes

Servings:4

Preparation Time: 5 minutes

Cooking Time: 10 minutes

Ingredients

For Cakes

- ½ a cup of coconut flour

- 2 tablespoon of Psyllium Husk powder
- ½ a teaspoon of garlic powder
- ¼ teaspoon of salt
- 2-3 scallions sliced up into thin portions
- ¼ cup of sesame oil
- 1 cup of warm water

For Sauce

- 1 tablespoon of tamari sauce
- 1 teaspoon of rice wine vinegar
- 1 tablespoon of water
- 1 teaspoon of sesame oil
- 1 finely minced garlic clove
- Chili flakes as needed

Directions:

1. Take a frying pan and place it over medium-

low heat

2. Add sesame oil and heat it up

3. Take a mixing bowl and add water, oil, garlic, salt, scallions, warm water and allow it to stand for 5 minutes to allow the flavors to mix up

4. Take another bowl and add coconut flour and the Psyllium Husk

5. Gently add the water to the dry ingredients, making sure to mix it well until the dough forms

6. Separate the dough into individual balls and flatten the balls into 4-inch rounds

7. Place the rounds in your skillet and fry for 5 minutes each side until they are golden

8. Keep repeating until the balls are used up

9. Enjoy!

Nutrition Values:

Calories: 206

Fat: 16G

Carbs: 4g

Protein: 4g

06. The Keto Crack Slaw

Servings:2

Preparation Time: 5 minutes

Cooking Time: 10 minutes

Ingredients

- 4 cups of shredded green cabbage
- ½ a cup of macadamia nuts chopped up
- 1 teaspoon of chili paste
- 1 teaspoon of vinegar
- 2 tablespoon of tamari

- 1 tablespoon of sesame oil
- 2 garlic cloves
- Sesame seeds as needed

Directions:

1. Take a pan and place it over medium-low heat and add tamari, sesame oil, vinegar, sesame oil, and chili paste
2. Add your green cabbage
3. Cover and allow it to cook for 5 minutes until the cabbage starts to tender
4. Stir everything and combine them well
5. Add the nuts
6. Cook for 5 minutes more until the nuts are tender
7. Serve and garnish

Enjoy!

Nutrition Values:

Calories: 360

Fat: 33g

Carbs: 7g

Protein: 7g

07. Feisty Grilled Artichokes

Preparation Time: 5 minutes

Cooking Time: 30 minute

Servings:4

Ingredients:

- 2 large sized artichokes
- 1 quartered lemon
- ¾ cup of extra virgin olive oil
- 4 chopped up garlic cloves
- 1 teaspoon of salt

- ½ a teaspoon of ground black pepper

Directions:

1. Take a large sized bowl and fill it up with cold water
2. Squeeze a bit of lemon juice from the wedges
3. Trim the upper part of your chokes, making sure to trim any damaged leaves as well
4. Cut the chokes up in half lengthwise portions
5. Add the chokes to your bowl of lemon water
6. Bring the whole pot to a boil
7. Pre-heat your outdoor grill to about medium-high heat
8. Allow the chokes to cook in the boiling pot for 15 minutes
9. Drain the chokes and keep them on the side
10. Take another medium-sized bowl and squeeze the remaining lemon

11. Stir in garlic and olive to the lemon mix
12. Brush up the chokes with the garlic dip and place them on your pre-heated grill
13. Grill for about 10 minutes, making sure to keep basting them until the edges are just slightly charred
14. Serve with the dip and enjoy!

Nutrition Values:

Calories: 402

Fat: 40g

Carbs: 10g

Protein: 2.9g

08. The Thundering Cinnamon Chocolate Smoothie

Servings:1

Preparation Time: 5 minutes

Cooking Time: 0 minutes

Ingredients

- ¾ cup of coconut milk
- ½ of a ripe avocado
- 2 teaspoon of unsweetened cocoa powder
- 1 teaspoon of cinnamon powder
- ¼ teaspoon of vanilla extract
- Stevia as needed
- ½ a teaspoon of coconut oil

Directions:

1. Add all of the ingredients to your blender and blend well until smooth
2. Allow them to chill and enjoy!

Nutrition Values:

Calories: 300

Fat: 30g

Carbs: 14g

Protein: 5g

09. Vegan Enchilada Macaroni

Servings:4

Preparation Time: 20 minutes

Cooking Time: 45 minutes

Ingredients

For Sauce

- 1 cup of hemp seeds
- ½ a cup of nutritional yeast
- ¼ cup of sliced red, yellow or orange bell peppers
- ½ a teaspoon of salt
- ½ a teaspoon of onion powder
- ½ a cup of water
- For The Main Recipe
- 2 pack of Shirataki macaroni (Tofu)

- 1 can of young, green jackfruit in brine
- ¼ cup of enchilada sauce

Directions:

1. Pre-heat your oven to a temperature of 350 degrees Fahrenheit
2. Drain and chop up your jackfruit with a knife and add 2 tablespoons of enchilada sauce, toss them well.
3. Keep it on the side
4. Blend the sauce ingredients in a blender and process them well
5. Drain and rinse the noodles thoroughly and transfer them to a baking dish
6. Add sauce, jackfruit to the baking dish and mix well
7. Bake for 45 minutes
8. Allow it to cool and enjoy!

Nutrition Values:

Calories: 192

Fat: 7.4g

Carbs: 4.1G

Protein: 9.6g

10. Squash Salad for the Green Lovers!

Preparation Time: 15 minutes

Cooking Time: 30 minutes

Servings:4

Ingredients:

- 2 tablespoons of extra virgin olive oil
- 1 small sized sliced onion
- 2 medium-sized coarsely chopped tomatoes
- 1 teaspoon of salt
- ¼ teaspoon of pepper

- 2 small zucchini cut up into ½ inch slices
- 2 small sized yellow summer squash cut up into ½ inch slices
- 1 bay leaf
- ½ a teaspoon of dried basil

Directions:

1. Take a skillet and place it over medium heat
2. Add oil and allow it to heat up
3. Add onions and stir-fry them for about 5 minutes
4. Add tomatoes to the pan and mix well
5. Season the mixture with salt and pepper
6. Keep stirring for about 5 minutes until nicely cooked
7. Add bay leaf, zucchini, yellow squash, and basil
8. Lower down the heat and allow it to simmer for

about 20 minutes, making sure to keep stirring it occasionally

9. Discard the bay leaf and enjoy!

Nutrition Values:

Calories: 65

Fat:5g

Carbs: 5g

Protein: 1.5G

11. Pumpkin Pecan Oatmeal

Preparation time: 10 minutes

Cooking time: 8 hours

Servings: 4

Ingredients:

- 1 and ½ cups water
- ½ cup pumpkin puree
- 1 teaspoon pumpkin pie spice

- 3 tablespoons stevia
- ½ cup steel cut oats
- ¼ cup pecans, chopped

Directions:

1. In your slow cooker mix water with oats, pumpkin puree, pumpkin spice, and stevia, stir, cover and cook on Low for 8 hours.
2. Sprinkle pecans on top, toss, divide into bowls and serve for breakfast.

Enjoy!

Nutrition Value: calories 211, fat 4, fiber 7, carbs 8, protein 3

12. Tasty Breakfast Burrito

Preparation time: 10 minutes

Cooking time: 6 hours

Servings: 8

Ingredients:

- 16 ounces tofu, crumbled
- 1 green bell pepper, chopped
- ¼ cup scallions, chopped
- 15 ounces canned black beans, drained
- 1 cup vegan salsa
- ½ cup of water
- ¼ teaspoon cumin, ground
- ½ teaspoon turmeric powder
- ½ teaspoon smoked paprika
- A pinch of salt and black pepper
- ¼ teaspoon chili powder
- 3 cups spinach leaves, torn
- 8 vegan tortillas for serving

Directions:

1. In your slow cooker, mix tofu with bell pepper, scallions, black beans, salsa, water, cumin, turmeric, paprika, salt, pepper, and chili powder, stir, cover and cook on Low for 6 hours.

2. Add spinach, toss well, divide this on your vegan tortillas, roll, wrap them and serve for breakfast.

3. Enjoy!

Nutrition Value: calories 211, fat 4, fiber 7, carbs 14, protein 4

13. Healthy Steel Cut Oats

Preparation time: 10 minutes

Cooking time: 4 hours

Servings: 6

Ingredients:

- 1 and ½ cups of water

- 1 and ½ cups of coconut milk
- 2 apples, cored, peeled and chopped
- 1 cup steel cut oats
- ½ teaspoon cinnamon powder
- ¼ teaspoon nutmeg, ground
- ¼ teaspoon allspice, ground
- ¼ teaspoon ginger powder
- ¼ teaspoon cardamom, ground
- 1 tablespoon flax seed, ground
- 2 teaspoons vanilla extract
- 2 teaspoons stevia
- Cooking spray

Directions:

1. Spray your slow cooker with cooking spray, add apple pieces, milk, water, cinnamon, oats,

allspice, nutmeg, cardamom, ginger, vanilla, flax seeds, and stevia, stir, cover and cook on Low for 4 hours.

2. Stir oatmeal again divides into bowls and serve.

Enjoy!

Nutrition Value: calories 162, fat 3, fiber 7, carbs 8, protein 5

14. Breakfast Tofu Casserole

Preparation time: 10 minutes

Cooking time: 4 hours

Servings: 4

Ingredients:

- 1 teaspoon lemon zest, grated
- 14 ounces tofu, cubed
- 1 tablespoon lemon juice
- 2 tablespoons nutritional yeast

- 1 tablespoon apple cider vinegar
- 1 tablespoon olive oil
- 2 garlic cloves, minced
- 10 ounces spinach, torn
- ½ cup yellow onion, chopped
- ½ teaspoon basil, dried
- 8 ounces mushrooms, sliced
- Salt and black pepper to the taste
- ¼ teaspoon red pepper flakes
- Cooking spray

Directions:

1. Spray your slow cooker with some cooking spray and arrange tofu cubes on the bottom.
2. Add lemon zest, lemon juice, yeast, vinegar, olive oil, garlic, spinach, onion, basil, mushrooms, salt, pepper, and pepper flakes,

toss, cover and cook on Low for 4 hours.

3. Divide between plates and serve for breakfast.

Enjoy!

Nutrition Value: calories 216, fat 6, fiber 8, carbs 12, protein 4

15. Carrot Oatmeal

Preparation time: 10 minutes

Cooking time: 7 hours

Servings: 4

Ingredients:

- 2 cups of coconut milk
- ½ cup steel cut oats
- 1 cup carrots, shredded
- 1 teaspoon cardamom, ground
- ½ teaspoon agave nectar
- A pinch of saffron

- Cooking spray

Directions:

1. Spray your slow cooker with cooking spray, add milk, oats, carrots, cardamom, and agave nectar, stir, cover and cook on Low for 7 hours.
2. Stir oatmeal again, divide into bowls, sprinkle saffron on top and serve for breakfast.
3. Enjoy!

Nutrition Value: calories 182, fat 7, fiber 4, carbs 8, protein 3

16. Delicious Vegan Scramble

Preparation time: 10 minutes

Cooking time: 8 hours

Servings: 4

Ingredients:

- 1 pound tofu, crumbled
- 1 pound white mushrooms, sliced

- 1 cup green onions, chopped
- 1 cup of corn
- 1 tablespoon olive oil
- A pinch of salt and black pepper
- 1 zucchini, chopped
- ¼ cup coconut aminos
- ½ cup nutritional yeast
- 3 pounds baby red potatoes, halved

Directions:

1. In your slow cooker, mix oil with tofu, mushrooms, green onions, corn, salt, pepper, zucchini, aminos, yeast and potatoes, toss, cover and cook on Low for 8 hours.
2. Divide between plates and serve for breakfast.

Enjoy!

Nutrition Value: calories 222, fat 5, fiber 8, carbs 12, protein 4

17. Blueberries Oatmeal

Preparation time: 10 minutes

Cooking time: 8 hours

Servings: 4

Ingredients:

- 1 cup blueberries
- 1 cup steel cut oats
- 1 cup of coconut milk
- 2 tablespoons agave nectar
- ½ teaspoon vanilla extract
- Coconut flakes for serving
- Cooking spray

Directions:

1. Spray your slow cooker with cooking spray, add

oats, milk, agave nectar, vanilla and blueberries, toss, cover and cook on Low for 8 hours.

2. Stir your oatmeal one more time, divide into bowls, sprinkle coconut flakes all over and serve.

Enjoy!

Nutrition Value: calories 182, fat 6, fiber 8, carbs 9, protein 6

18. Sweet Apple And Pears Breakfast

Preparation time: 10 minutes

Cooking time: 6 hours

Servings: 6

Ingredients:

- 4 apples, cored, peeled and cut into medium chunks
- 1 teaspoon lemon juice

- 4 pears, cored, peeled and cut into medium chunks
- 5 teaspoons stevia
- 1 teaspoon cinnamon powder
- 1 teaspoon vanilla extract
- ½ teaspoon ginger, ground
- ½ teaspoon cloves, ground
- ½ teaspoon cardamom, ground

Directions:

1. In your slow cooker, mix apples with pears, lemon juice, stevia, cinnamon, vanilla extract, ginger, cloves, and cardamom, stir, cover and cook on Low for 6 hours.
2. Divide into bowls and serve for breakfast.

Enjoy!

Nutrition Value: calories 201, fat 3, fiber 7, carbs 19, protein 4

19. Almond Butter Oatmeal

Preparation time: 10 minutes

Cooking time: 10 hours

Servings: 2

Ingredients:

- ½ cup steel cut oats
- ½ cup almond milk
- Seeds from 1 vanilla bean
- 1 cup of water
- 4 tablespoons almond butter
- Stevia to the taste

Directions:

1. In 2 heatproof containers, divide oats, almond milk, vanilla seeds, water, stevia, and almond butter and stir.

2. Arrange containers in your slow cooker, fill slow cooker halfway with water, cover and cook on Low for 10 hours.
3. Serve warm for breakfast.

Enjoy!

Nutrition Value: calories 182, fat 3, fiber 7, carbs 18, protein 4

20. Banana Oatmeal

Preparation time: 10 minutes

Cooking time: 8 hours

Servings: 4

Ingredients:

- 1 banana, peeled and mashed
- 1 cup steel cut oats
- 2 cups almond milk
- 2 cups of water

- ¼ cup walnuts, chopped
- 2 tablespoons flax seed meal
- 2 teaspoons cinnamon powder
- 1 teaspoon vanilla extract
- ½ teaspoon nutmeg, ground

Directions:

1. In your slow cooker mix oats with almond milk, water, walnuts, flaxseed meal, cinnamon, vanilla, and nutmeg, stir, cover and cook on Low for 8 hours.
2. Stir oatmeal one more time, divide into bowls and serve for breakfast.

Enjoy!

Nutrition Value: calories 291, fat 7, fiber 6, carbs 42, protein 11

21. Delicious Vegan Frittata

Preparation time: 10 minutes

Cooking time: 6 hours

Servings: 4

Ingredients:

- 1 pound firm tofu, drained, pressed and crumbled
- 2 tablespoons olive oil
- ¼ cup nutritional yeast
- 1 yellow onion, chopped
- ¼ teaspoon turmeric powder
- 3 tablespoons garlic, minced
- 1 red bell pepper, chopped
- ½ cup kalamata olives pitted and halved
- 1 teaspoon basil, dried
- 1 teaspoon oregano, dried
- 1 tablespoon lemon juice

- Salt and black pepper to the taste

Directions:

1. Add the oil to your slow cooker and arrange crumbled tofu on the bottom.

2. Add yeast, onion, turmeric, garlic, bell pepper, olives, basil, oregano, lemon juice, salt, and pepper, toss a bit, cover and cook on Low for 6 hours.

3. Divide frittata between plates and serve for breakfast.

Enjoy!

Nutrition Value: calories 271, fat 4, fiber 7, carbs 20, protein 6

22. Apple Granola

Preparation time: 10 minutes

Cooking time: 4 hours

Servings: 3

Ingredients:

- ½ cup granola
- ½ cup bran flakes
- 2 green apples, cored, peeled and roughly chopped
- ¼ cup apple juice
- 1/8 cup maple syrup
- 2 tablespoons cashew butter
- 1 teaspoon cinnamon powder
- ½ teaspoon nutmeg, ground

Directions:

- In your slow cooker, mix granola with bran flakes, apples, apple juice, maple syrup, cashew butter, cinnamon, and nutmeg, toss, cover and cook on Low for 4 hours.
- Divide apple granola into bowls and serve for breakfast.

Enjoy!

Nutrition Value: calories 218, fat 6, fiber 9, carbs 17, protein 6

23. Carrot And Zucchini Oatmeal

Preparation time: 10 minutes

Cooking time: 8 hours

Servings: 4

Ingredients:

- ½ cup steel cut oats
- 1 carrot, grated
- 1 and ½ cups of almond milk
- ¼ zucchini, grated
- A pinch of nutmeg, ground
- A pinch of cloves, ground
- ½ teaspoon cinnamon powder
- 2 tablespoons maple syrup

- ¼ cup pecans, chopped
- 1 teaspoon vanilla extract

Directions:

1. In your slow cooker, mix oats with carrot, zucchini, almond milk, cloves, nutmeg, cinnamon, maple syrup, pecans, and vanilla extract, stir, cover and cook on Low for 8 hours.
2. Stir your oatmeal one more time, divide into bowls and serve.

Enjoy!

Nutrition Value: calories 215, fat 4, fiber 7, carbs 12, protein 7

24. Cranberry Breakfast Quinoa

Preparation time: 10 minutes

Cooking time: 2 hours

Servings: 4

Ingredients:

- 1 cup quinoa
- 3 cups of coconut water
- 1 teaspoon vanilla extract
- 3 teaspoons stevia
- 1/8 cup coconut flakes
- ¼ cup cranberries, dried
- 1/8 cup almonds, chopped

Directions:

1. In your slow cooker, mix quinoa with coconut water, vanilla, stevia, coconut flakes, almonds and cranberries, toss, cover and cook on High for 2 hours.
2. Stir quinoa mix one more time, divide into bowls and serve for breakfast.

Enjoy!

Nutrition Value: calories 246, fat 5, fiber 5, carbs 30, protein 7

25. Delicious Quinoa And Oats

Preparation time: 10 minutes

Cooking time: 7 hours

Servings: 6

Ingredients:

- ½ cup quinoa
- 1 and ½ cups steel cut oats
- 4 tablespoons stevia
- 4 and ½ cups of almond milk
- 2 tablespoons maple syrup
- 1 and ½ teaspoons vanilla extract
- Strawberries halved for serving
- Cooking spray

Directions:

1. Spray your slow cooker with cooking spray, add oats, quinoa, stevia, almond milk, maple syrup, and vanilla extract, toss, cover and cook on Low for 7 hours.

2. Divide into bowls, add strawberries on top, and serve for breakfast.

Enjoy!

Nutrition Value: calories 267, fat 5, fiber 8, carbs 28, protein 5

26. Breakfast Chia Pudding

Preparation time: 10 minutes

Cooking time: 2 hours

Servings: 4

Ingredients:

- ½ cup coconut chia granola
- ½ cup chia seeds

- 2 cups of coconut milk
- 2 tablespoons coconut, shredded and unsweetened
- ¼ cup maple syrup
- ½ teaspoon cinnamon powder
- 2 teaspoons cocoa powder
- ½ teaspoon vanilla extract

Directions:

1. In your slow cooker, mix chia granola with chia seeds, coconut milk, coconut, maple syrup, cinnamon, cocoa powder, and vanilla, toss, cover and cook on High for 2 hours.
2. Divide chia pudding into bowls and serve for breakfast.

Enjoy!

Nutrition Value: calories 261, fat 4, fiber 8, carbs 10, protein 4

MAINS

27. Stinky Roasted Garlic

Servings: 2

Preparation Time: 5 minutes

Cooking Time: 20 minutes

Ingredients

- 2 medium garlic heads
- 2 tablespoon of olive oil

Directions

- Pre-heat your oven to a temperature of 250 degrees Fahrenheit
- Peel each of your garlic clove
- Place the cloves in a single layer in a small sized baking dish and drizzle some olive oil
- Bake for about 15 minutes until the garlic are tender

Nutrition Value:

Calories: 81

Fat: 7g

Carbs: 5g

Protein: 1G

28. The Crazy Tofu Bok Choy Salad

Servings:5

Preparation Time: 30 minutes

Cooking Time: 30 minutes

Ingredients

Oven Baked Tofu

- 15 ounces of extra firm tofu
- 1 tablespoon of Tamari
- 1 tablespoon of sesame oil
- 1 tablespoon of water
- 2 teaspoon of minced garlic

- 1 tablespoon of rice wine vinegar
- ½ a lemon juice

Bok Choy Salad

- 9 ounces of Bok Choy
- 1 green onion stalk
- 2 tablespoon of chopped cilantro
- 3 tablespoon of coconut oil
- 2 tablespoon of Tamari
- 1 tablespoon of Sambal Olek
- 1 tablespoon of peanut butter
- Juice of ½ a lime
- 7 drops of liquid Stevia

Directions

1. Press your tofu with heavy weight for 5 hours
2. Take a bowl and add all of the marinade

ingredients - Tamari, water, sesame oil, garlic, lemon juice, and vinegar

3. Chop up the tofu into square pieces and place them in a bag alongside the marinade
4. Allow them to marinate for 30 minutes or overnight
5. Pre-heat your oven to 350 degrees Fahrenheit and place your tofu on a baking sheet lined up the parchment paper
6. Bake for 30-35 minutes
7. Add all of the salad dressing mixtures except Bok Choy in a bowl and mix well
8. Add chopped up Bok Choy
9. Toss well
10. Remove the tofu from your oven and assemble the salad by mixing the Bok Choy, Tofu, and Sauce

Enjoy!

Nutrition Values:

Calories: 398

Fat: 30g

Carbs: 6g

Protein: 24g

29. A Spicy Red Coconut Curry for Keto Vegans

Servings:4

Preparation Time: 10 minutes

Cooking Time: 25 minutes

Ingredients

- 1 cup of broccoli florets
- 1 large sized handful of spinach
- 4 tablespoon of coconut oil
- ¼ medium onion

- 1 teaspoon of minced garlic
- 1 teaspoon of minced ginger
- 2 teaspoon of Tamari
- 1 tablespoon of red curry paste
- ½ a cup of coconut cream
- 2 teaspoon of special sauce

Special Sauce

- 1 and a ½ cup of shredded seaweed
- 6 cups of water
- 6 fat clove garlic crushed but not peeled
- 1 tablespoon of peppercorns
- 1 cup of mushroom Tamari
- 1 tablespoon of miso

Directions

1. Take a large saucepan and add garlic,

peppercorns, water and bring to a boil

2. Lower down the heat and simmer for 20 minutes
3. Strain and return the liquid to the pot
4. Add Tamari and bring to a boil again and cook it is very salty
5. Remove the heat and stir in miso
6. This is your special sauce
7. Chop up your onion and mince garlic
8. Take a pan and place it over medium-high heat, add chopped up onions and minced garlic
9. Add two tablespoon of coconut oil and cook until translucent
10. Turn the heat down to medium-low and add broccoli to the pan, stir well
11. Once the broccoli is cooked, move the veggies on the side and add curry paste

12. Cook for 60 seconds

13. Add spinach and top and cook until wilt, add coconut cream alongside the remaining coconut oil

14. Stir and add Tamari, special sauce, ginger and allow it to simmer for 10 minutes more

Enjoy!

Nutrition Values:

Calories: 310

Fat: 22G

Carbs: 5g

Protein: 25G

30. Quick and Easy Caesar Salad

Servings:4

Preparation Time: 10 minutes

Cooking Time: 0 minutes

Ingredients

- 1 piece of ripe avocado
- 3 tablespoon of lemon juice
- 2 tablespoon of water
- 3 minced garlic minced up
- 1 tablespoon of caper brine
- 1 tablespoon of capers
- 2 teaspoon of Dijon mustard
- Sea salt as needed
- Pepper as needed
- ¼ cup of hemp seeds
- 12 cups of chopped up romaine leaves

Directions

1. Take a bowl and add avocado, water, lemon juice, brine, garlic, capers, pepper and mustard salt

2. Add the contents to a blender and pulse until smooth
3. Add some water if your desired consistency is not reached
4. Spoon the dressing into a bowl
5. Add hemp seeds and mix
6. Add romaine lettuce to a large sized salad bowl and drop the dressing on top

Enjoy!

Nutrition Values:

Calories: 281

Fat: 24g

Carbs: 12G

Protein: 6g

31. Creamy Roasted Pepper Soup

Servings:4

Preparation Time: 0 minutes

Cooking Time: 30 minutes

Ingredients

- 2 tablespoon of coconut butter
- ½ a cup of roasted red pepper chopped up
- 1 large sized finely chopped shallots
- 1 teaspoon of celery salt
- 1 tablespoon of seasoned salt
- 1 teaspoon of organic paprika
- 1 pinch of crushed red pepper flakes
- 4-5 cups of Cauliflower broken up into florets
- 4 cup of vegetable broth
- Just a splash of apple cider vinegar
- 1 pinch fresh thyme
- 1 cup of organic coconut milk

Directions

1. Take a heavy bottomed pot and add coconut oil over medium heat
2. Add chopped up shallots and Saute for 3 minutes
3. Add chopped up and roasted pepper alongside the seasonings
4. Stir well and cook for 2-3 minutes
5. Add cauliflower, fresh thyme, and stock
6. Bring it to a simmer and cover the pot, cook for 5-10 minutes
7. Work in small batches and puree the soup using an immersion blender
8. Bring back the whole blended soup back to your pot and stir in coconut milk

Enjoy!

Nutrition Values:

Calories: 171

Fat: 16G

Carbs: 7g

Protein: 1G

32. Spiralized Asian Zucchini Salad

Servings:10

Preparation Time: 10 minutes

Cooking Time: 0 minutes

Ingredients

- 1 thinly spiralized medium zucchini
- 1 pound of shredded cabbage
- 1 cup of sunflower seeds
- 1 cup of sliced almonds
- ¾ cup of avocado oil

- 1/3 cup of white vinegar
- 1 teaspoon of Stevia

Directions

1. Cut up the spiralized zucchini into small portions using a kitchen knife
2. Take a large sized bowl and add sunflower seeds, cabbage, and almonds
3. Stir in zucchini
4. Take a small sized bowl and add oil, Stevia, and vinegar
5. Pour the dressing on top of the veggies and stir well
6. Chill for 2 hours and

enjoy!

Nutrition Values:

Calories: 120

Fat: 10g

Carbs: 7g

Protein: 4g

33. Forever Together Courgette Salad

Preparation Time: 20 minutes

Cooking Time: No cook required

Servings:2

Ingredients

- Juice of 1 lemon
- 2 tablespoons of extra virgin olive oil
- ½ of a small pack of chopped up chives
- ½ of a small chopped up mint
- 300g of courgettes

Directions:

1. Take a large-sized bowl and pour lemon juice
2. Season with some salt and pepper

3. Whisk in olive oil and add the chopped up herbs
4. Put Courgette through a Spiralizer using the noodle attachment
5. Tip the zoodles to your bowl
6. Add the prepped salad dressing
7. Toss everything well
8. Serve and enjoy!

Nutrition Values:

Calories: 144

Fat: 12G

Carbs: 4g

Protein: 4g

34. Roasted Cauliflower Soup

Servings: 6

Preparation Time: 15 minutes

Cooking Time: 60 minutes

Ingredients

- 2 cauliflower head broken up into florets
- Olive oil cooking spray
- ¼ cup of olive oil
- 1 chopped up a large onion
- 4 cloves of chopped up garlic
- 6 cups of water
- Salt as needed
- Pepper as needed

Directions

1. Add cauliflower florets to a large-sized bowl filled with salty water, wait for 20 minutes
2. Drain and arrange them on a sheet of aluminum foil on your baking sheet
3. Spray olive oil evenly over the cauliflower

4. Pre-heat your broiler to high and set the rack 6 inch away from the heat source
5. Broil for 20-30 minutes
6. Take a large soup pot and place it over medium heat
7. Add onion and cook for 5 minutes
8. Stir in garlic, roasted cauliflower and water and cook for 30 minutes
9. Blend the soup using an immersion blender and serve!

Nutrition Value:

Calories: 140

Fat: 10g

Carbs: 11G

Protein: 6g

35. Fine Vegan Pad Thai of Very Low Carb

Servings:4

Preparation Time: 15 minutes

Cooking Time: 20 minutes

Ingredients

- 1 bag of Kelp noodles
- ½ cup of peanut butter
- 1 medium-sized white onion
- ¼ cup of Tamari
- Juice of 1 lime
- 3 cloves of garlic
- 2 teaspoon of red pepper flakes
- Shredded up carrots, chopped scallions, sesame seeds, and cilantro

Directions

1. Soak your noodles under water and allow them to wilt
2. Take a food processor and add peanut butter,

tamari, onion, lime juice, garlic, and pepper flakes

3. Process well
4. Drain the noodles and add ¼ of the sauce on top of the noodles
5. Give the whole mixture a toss
6. Serve with garnish and enjoy!

Nutrition Values:

Calories: 231

Fat: 16G

Carbs: 7g

Protein: 7g

36. Vegan White Pizza

Preparation Time: 15 MINUTES

Servings: 2

Ingredients:

- 1 store-bought Pizza Crust
- ¼ cup Vegan Alfredo Sauce
- 1 tsp chopped Oregano
- ½ cup shredded Vegan Cheese
- 1 ½ cups Water

Directions:

1. Pour the water into your IP. Lower the trivet.
2. Line a baking dish that can fit into the IP with parchment paper.
3. Roll out the pizza crust and place inside the baking dish.
4. Spread the Alfredo sauce over the crust and sprinkle the cheese over.
5. Top with chopped oregano.
6. Place the dish on the lowered trivet and close the lid of the IP.

7. Set the IP to MANUAL and cook the pizza for 5 minutes on HIGH.
8. Do a quick pressure release.
9. Serve and enjoy!

Nutrition Value:

Calories 390

Total Fats 20g

Carbs 30g

Protein 8g

Fiber: 2G

37. Mini Vegan Shephard's Pie

Preparation Time: 20 MINUTES

Servings: 4

Ingredients:

- 1 cup diced Onion
- 2 cups steamed and Mashed Cauliflower

- 1 cup grated Potatoes
- 1 cup diced Tomatoes
- 1 ½ cup Water

Directions:

α. Add a splash of water to your IP and set it to SAUTE.

β. Add the onions and cook for 2 minutes.

χ. Add the potatoes and cook on SAUTE for 5 minutes, stirring frequently.

δ. Stir in the tomatoes and cook for 3 more minutes.

ε. Divide the mixture between 4 greased ramekins.

ϕ. Top with the mashed potatoes.

γ. Pour the water into the IP and lower the trivet.

η. Place the ramekins on the trivet and close the

lid.

ι. Cook on HIGH for 5 minutes.

φ. Serve and enjoy!

Nutrition Value:

Calories 225

Total Fats 14g

Carbs 5g

Protein 12G

Fiber: 0.3g

38. Mushroom Pasta

Preparation Time: 20 MINUTES

Servings: 4

Ingredients:

- 1 ½ cups sliced Mushrooms
- 1 cup Coconut Milk

- 2 cups Water
- 1 tsp Arrowroot
- 2 cups Pasta, uncooked

Directions:

1. Add a splash of the coconut milk in the IP and set it to SAUTE.
2. Add mushrooms and cook for a few minutes.
3. Stir in the rest of the milk, water, and pasta.
4. Close the lid and set the IP to MANUAL.
5. Cook on HIGH for 7 minutes.
6. Do a quick pressure release and set the IP to SAUTE.
7. Whisk in the arrowroot and cook until the sauce thickens a bit.
8. Serve and enjoy!

Nutrition Value:

Calories 452

Total Fats 15G

Carbs 34g

Protein 15G

Fiber: 3g

39. Basil Risotto

Preparation Time: 30 MINUTES

Servings: 6

Ingredients:

- 1 ½ tbsp Olive Oil
- 1 Onion, chopped
- 28 ounces Vegetable Broth
- 12 ounces Arborio Rice
- 1 ½ cups chopped Basil

Directions:

1. Heat the oil in the IP on SAUTE.
2. Add the onions and cook for 3 minutes.
3. Add the rice and cook for another minute.
4. Pour the broth over, give it a stir, and close the lid.
5. Cook on RICE for 15 minutes.
6. Do a quick pressure release.
7. Stir in the basil and cook on SAUTE for another minute.
8. Serve and enjoy!

Nutrition Value:

Calories 260

Total Fats 5g

Carbs 46g

Protein 7.8g

Fiber: 2G

40. Vegan Cheese and Asparagus Pasta

Preparation Time: 20 MINUTES

Servings: 4

Ingredients:

- 1 cup shredded Vegan Cheese
- 2 cups Pasta
- 6 Asparagus Spears, chopped
- ½ cup Vegan Alfredo Sauce
- 3 ½ cups Veggie Broth

Directions:

1. Combine the pasta, asparagus, and broth, in the IP.
2. Close the lid and set it to MANUAL.
3. Cook on HIGH for 7 minutes.
4. Release the pressure quickly.

5. Drain the pasta and return it to the IP.
6. Stir in the sauce and cheese.
7. Cook on SAUTE for 2 minutes.
8. Serve and enjoy!

Nutrition Value:

Calories 480

Total Fats 12G

Carbs 39g

Protein 8g

Fiber: 2G

41. Carrot and Sweet Potato Medley

Preparation Time: 20 MINUTES

Servings: 4

Ingredients:

1. 2 tbsp Olive Oil
2. 2 pounds Sweet Potatoes, cubed

3. 1 Onion, chopped
4. 2 pounds Baby Carrots, halved
5. 1 cup Veggie Broth

Directions:

1. Heat the oil in your IP on SAUTE.
2. Add the onion and cook until soft, about 5 minutes.
3. Add the remaining ingredients, stir to combine, and close the lid.
4. Set the IP to MANUAL and cook on HIGH for 8 minutes.
5. Release the pressure quickly.
6. Serve and enjoy!

Nutrition Value:

Calories 413

Total Fats 7.5g

Carbs 76g

Protein 7g

Fiber: 13G

42. Pesto Farfale

Preparation Time: 10 MINUTES

Servings: 4

Ingredients:

1. 12 ounces Farfale
2. ¾ cup Vegan Pesto
3. 4 cups Water
4. 1 cup Cherry Tomatoes

Directions:

1. Combine the farfalle and water in your IP.
2. Close the lid and set the pot to MANUAL.
3. Cook on HIGH for 7 minutes.
4. Do a quick pressure release.

5. Drain the pasta and return to the pot.
6. Stir in the pesto sauce and cook on SAUTE for 1 more minute.
7. Quarter the cherry tomatoes and stir into the pasta.
8. Serve and enjoy!

Nutrition Value:

Calories 390

Total Fats 9g

Carbs 40g

Protein 8g

Fiber: 1G

43. Mexican Rice Casserole

Preparation Time: 35 MINUTES

Servings: 4

Ingredients:

- 1 cup Black Beans, soaked overnight and drained
- 5 cups Water
- 2 cups Brown Rice
- 6 ounces Salsa Paste
- 2 tsp Cumin

Directions:

1. Combine all of the ingredients in your Instant Pot.
2. Close the lid and set the IP to MANUAL.
3. Cook on HIGH for 28 minutes.
4. Do a quick pressure release.
5. Serve garnished with lime and cilantro, if desired.
6. Enjoy!

Nutrition Value:

Calories 322

Total Fats 2G

Carbs 60 g

Protein 6g

Fiber: 8g

44. Warm Collard Salad

Preparation Time: 5 minutes

Cooking Time: 5 minutes

Serving Size: 2

Ingredients

- ¾ cup coconut whipping cream
- 2 tbsp vegan mayonnaise
- A pinch of mustard powder
- 2 tbsp coconut oil

- 1 garlic clove, minced
- Salt and freshly ground black pepper
- 2 oz. vegan butter
- 1 cup collards, rinsed
- 4 oz. tofu cheese

Directions

1. In a small bowl, whisk the coconut whipping cream, vegan mayonnaise, mustard powder, coconut oil, garlic, salt, and black pepper until well mixed; set aside.
2. Melt the vegan butter in a large skillet over medium heat and sauté the collards until wilted and brownish. Season with salt and black pepper to taste.
3. Transfer the collards to a salad bowl and pour the creamy dressing over. Mix the salad well and crumble the tofu cheese over.
4. Serve the salad immediately with cauli

couscous.

Nutrition Value:

Calories: 495; Total Fat: 46g; Total Carbs: 8g; Fiber: 3g; Net Carbs: 5g; Protein: 11G

45. Fried Broccoli Salad with Tempeh and Cranberries

Preparation Time: 5 minutes

Cooking Time: 6 minutes

Serving Size: 4

Ingredients

- 3 oz. vegan butter
- ¾ lb tempeh slices, cut into 1-inch cubes
- 1 lb broccoli florets
- Salt and ground black pepper to taste
- 2 oz. almonds
- ½ cup frozen cranberries

Directions

1. In a deep skillet, melt the vegan butter over medium heat until no longer foaming, and fry the tempeh cubes until brown on all sides.

2. Add the broccoli and stir-fry for 6 minutes. Season with salt and pepper. Turn the heat off. Stir in the almonds and cranberries to warm through. Share the salad into four bowls and serve.

Nutrition Value:

Calories: 740; Total Fat: 72G; Total Carbs: 12G; Fiber: 5g; Net Carbs: 7g; Protein: 12G

46. Tangy Nutty Brussel Sprout Salad

Preparation Time: 13 minutes

Cooking Time: 4 minutes

Serving Size: 4

Ingredients

- 1 lb Brussels sprouts, trimmed

- 1 lemon, juice and zest
- ½ cup olive oil
- Salt and pepper to taste
- Spicy pecans and seed mix
- 1 tbsp vegan butter
- 1 tsp chili paste
- 2 oz. pecans
- 1 oz. pumpkin seeds
- 1 oz. sunflower seeds
- ½ tsp cumin powder
- 1 pinch salt

Directions

1. Place the Brussels sprouts in a food processor and shred coarsely. Transfer to a salad bowl.
2. In a small bowl, mix the lemon juice, zest, olive

oil, salt, and pepper, and drizzle the dressing over the Brussels sprouts. Toss and allow the vegetable to marinate for 10 minutes.

3. Meanwhile, melt the vegan butter in a frying pan. Stir in the chili and then, toss the pecans, pumpkin seeds, sunflower seeds, cumin powder, and salt in the chili butter.

4. Sauté on low heat for 3 to 4 minutes just to heat the nuts but not exude the flavor. Turn the heat off and allow cooling. Pour the nuts and seeds mix in the salad bowl, toss, and enjoy the salad.

Nutrition Value:

Calories: 420; Total Fat: 35g; Total Carbs: 15G; Fiber: 7g; Net Carbs: 8g; Protein: 12G

ENTREES

47. Tomato Cream Soup with Basil

Preparation Time: 20 minutes

Servings: 2-4

Ingredients

- 1 carrot, chopped
- 2 tbsp olive oil
- 1 onion, diced
- 1 garlic clove, minced
- ¼ cup raw cashew nuts, diced
- 14 ounces canned tomatoes
- 1 tsp fresh basil leaves + extra to garnish
- 1 cup of water
- Salt and black pepper to taste
- 1 cup crème fraîche

Directions

1. Warm olive oil in a pot over medium heat and sauté the onion, carrot, and garlic for 4 minutes until softened. Stir in the tomatoes, basil, water, cashew nuts, and season with salt and black pepper.

2. Cover and bring to simmer for 10 minutes until thoroughly cooked. Puree the ingredients with an immersion blender. Adjust to taste and stir in the crème fraîche. Serve sprinkled with basil.

Nutrition Value:

Calories: 253, Fat: 23.5G, Net Carbs: 6.2G, Protein: 4.1G

48. Vegan Coconut Green Soup

Preparation Time: 30 minutes

Servings: 2-4

Ingredients

- 1 broccoli head, chopped
- 1 cup spinach

- 1 onion, chopped
- 1 garlic clove, minced
- ½ cup leeks
- 3 cups vegetable stock
- ½ cup of coconut milk
- 2 tbsp coconut oil
- 1 bay leaf
- Salt and black pepper, to taste
- 2 tbsp coconut yogurt

Directions

1. Warm coconut oil in a large pot over medium heat. Add onion, leeks, and garlic and cook for 5 minutes. Add broccoli and cook for an additional 5 minutes. Pour in the stock over and add the bay leaf. Close the lid, bring to a boil, and reduce the heat. Simmer for about 10 minutes.

2. Add spinach and cook for 3 more minutes. Discard the bay leaf and blend the soup with a hand blender. Stir in the coconut cream, salt, and black pepper. Divide among serving bowls and garnish with a swirl of coconut yogurt.

Nutrition Value:

Calories: 272, Fat:: 24.5g, Net Carbs:: 4.3g, Protein:: 4.5g

49. Hearty Vegetable Soup

Preparation Time: 25 minutes

Servings: 2-4

Ingredients

- 2 tsp olive oil
- 1 onion, chopped
- 1 garlic clove, minced
- ½ celery stalk, chopped
- 1 cup mushrooms, sliced

- ½ head broccoli, chopped
- ½ carrot, sliced
- 1 cup spinach, torn into pieces
- Salt and black pepper, to taste
- 2 thyme sprigs, chopped
- 3 cups vegetable stock
- 1 tomato, chopped
- ½ cup almond milk

Directions

1. Heat olive oil in a saucepan. Add onion, celery, garlic, and carrot; sauté until translucent, occasionally stirring, about 5 minutes.
2. Place in spinach, mushrooms, salt, rosemary, tomatoes, bay leaves, black pepper, thyme, and vegetable stock. Simmer the mixture for 15 minutes while the lid is slightly open.

3. Stir in almond milk and cook for 5 more minutes.

Nutrition Value:

Calories: 167; Fat:: 6.2G, Net Carbs:: 7.9g, Protein:: 3.2G

50. Vegan Cream Soup with Avocado & Zucchini

Preparation Time: 35 minutes

Servings: 2

Ingredients

- 3 tsp vegetable oil
- 1 leek, chopped
- 1 rutabaga, sliced
- 3 cups zucchinis, chopped
- 1 avocado, chopped
- Salt and black pepper to taste
- 4 cups vegetable broth

- 2 tbsp fresh mint, chopped

Directions

1. In a pot, sauté leek, zucchini, and rutabaga in warm oil for about 7-10 minutes. Season with black pepper and salt. Pour in broth and bring to a boil. Lower the heat and simmer for 20 minutes.

2. Lift from the heat. In batches, add the soup and avocado to a blender. Blend until creamy and smooth. Serve in bowls topped with fresh mint.

Nutrition Value:

Calories: 378 Fat:: 24.5g, Net Carbs:: 9.3g, Protein:: 8.2G

51. Mediterranean Artichoke & Red Onion Salad

Preparation Time: 30 minutes

Servings: 2

Ingredients

- 6 baby artichoke hearts, halved

- ½ lemon, juiced
- ½ red onion, sliced
- ¼ cup cherry peppers halved
- ¼ cup pitted olives, sliced
- ¼ cup olive oil
- ¼ tsp lemon zest
- 2 tsp balsamic vinegar, sugar-free
- 1 tbsp chopped dill
- Salt and black pepper to taste
- 1 tbsp capers

Directions

1. Bring a pot of salted water to a boil. Add the artichokes to the pot. lower the heat, and let simmer for 20 minutes until tender. Drain and place the artichokes in a bowl.
2. Add in the rest of the ingredients, except for

the olives; toss to combine well. Transfer to a serving platter and top with the olives.

Nutrition Value:

Calories: 464, Fat:: 31.2G, Net Carbs:: 9.5g, Protein:: 13.4g

52. Fresh Avocado-Cucumber Soup

Preparation Time: 10 minutes + chilling time

Servings: 2-4

Ingredients

- 3 tbsp olive oil
- 1 small onion, chopped
- 4 large cucumbers, seeded, chopped
- 1 large avocado, peeled and pitted
- Salt and black pepper to taste
- 1 ½ cups water
- ½ cup Greek yogurt

- 1 tbsp cilantro, chopped
- 2 limes, juiced
- 1 garlic clove, minced
- 2 tomatoes, chopped
- 1 chopped avocado for garnish

Directions

- Pour all the ingredient, except for the tomatoes and avocado in the food processor. Puree the ingredients for 2 minutes or until smooth. Pour the mixture in a bowl. Cover and refrigerate for 2 hours. Top with avocado and tomatoes.

Nutrition Value:

Calories: 343, Fat: 26.4g, Net Carbs: 5.3g, Protein: 10g

53. Almond Parsnip Soup

Preparation Time: 25 minutes

Servings: 2-4

Ingredients

- 1 tbsp olive oil
- 1 cup onion, chopped
- 1 celery, chopped
- 2 cloves garlic, minced
- 2 turnips, peeled and chopped
- 4 cups vegetable broth
- Salt and white pepper, to taste
- ¼ cup ground almonds
- 1 cup almond milk
- 1 tbsp fresh cilantro, chopped

Directions

1. Warm the oil in a pot over medium heat and sauté celery, garlic, and onion for 6 minutes. Stir in white pepper, broth, salt, and ground almonds. Boil the mixture.

2. Bring to the boil and simmer for 15 minutes. Transfer the soup to an immersion blender and puree. Serve garnished with sour cream and cilantro.

Nutrition Value:

Calories: 125; Fat:: 7.1g, Net Carbs:: 7.7g, Protein:: 4g

54. Sauteed Spinach with Spicy Tofu

Preparation Time: 25 minutes

Servings: 2-4

Ingredients

- 2 tbsp olive oil
- 14 ounces block tofu, pressed and cubed
- 1 celery stalk, chopped
- 1 bunch scallions, chopped
- 1 tsp cayenne pepper
- 1 tsp garlic powder

- 2 tbsp Worcestershire sauce
- Salt and black pepper, to taste
- 1 pound spinach, chopped
- ½ tsp turmeric powder
- ¼ tsp dried basil

Directions

1. In a large skillet over medium heat, warm 1 tablespoon of olive oil. Stir in tofu cubes and cook for 8 minutes. Place in scallions and celery; cook for 5 minutes until soft. Stir in cayenne, Worcestershire sauce, black pepper, salt, and garlic; cook for 3 more minutes; set aside.

2. In the same pan, warm the remaining 1 tablespoon of oil. Add in spinach and the remaining seasonings and cook for 4 minutes. Mix in tofu mixture and serve warm.

Nutrition Value:

Calories: 205; Fat:: 12.5g, Net Carbs:: 7.8g, Protein:: 7.7g

55. Cauliflower & Celery Bisque

Preparation Time: 30 minutes

Servings: 2-4

Ingredients

- 2 tbsp olive oil
- 1 onion, finely chopped
- 1 garlic clove, minced
- 1 head cauliflower, cut into florets
- ½ cup celery, chopped
- 4 cups vegetable broth
- ½ cup heavy cream
- Salt and black pepper to taste
- 1 tbsp parsley, chopped

Directions

1. Set a large pot over medium heat and warm the olive oil. Add celery, garlic, and onion and sauté until translucent, about 5 minutes. Place in vegetable broth, and cauliflower.

2. Bring to a boil, reduce the heat and simmer for 15-20 minutes. Transfer the soup to an immersion blender and blend to achieve the required consistency; top with parsley to serve.

Nutrition Value:

Calories: 187; Fat:: 13.5g, Net Carbs:: 5.6g, Protein:: 4.1G

56. Crunchy Rosemary Almonds

Preparation Time: 10 minutes

Servings: 4

Ingredients:

- 2 cups almonds
- 1 tsp smoked paprika

- 2 tbsp olive oil
- 2 tbsp rosemary, sliced
- 1 tsp salt

Directions:

1. Heat olive oil in a pan over medium-high heat.
2. Once the oil is hot, then add almonds and cook for 3 minutes.
3. Season almonds with paprika, rosemary, and salt.
4. Serve and enjoy.

Nutrition Value:

Calories 342

Fat 31 g

Carbs 11 g

Sugar 2 g

Protein 10 g

Cholesterol 0 mg

57. Simple Cauliflower Popcorn

Preparation Time: 50 minutes

Servings: 4

Ingredients:

- 1 large cauliflower head, cut into florets
- 2 tbsp butter, melted
- 2 tbsp coconut oil, melted
- Salt

Directions:

- Preheat the oven to 400 F.
- Add cauliflower florets into the bowl.
- Pour melted coconut oil and butter all over cauliflower florets.
- Season with salt and toss well.
- Place cauliflower florets on baking sheet and

roast in preheated oven for 40 minutes. Stir after every 15 minutes.

- Serve and enjoy.

Nutrition Value:
Calories 162

Fat 12 g

Carbs 11 g

Sugar 5 g

Protein 4 g

Cholesterol 15 mg

58. Healthy Avocado Fries

Preparation Time: 30 minutes

Servings: 4

Ingredients:

- 2 avocado, chopped into wedges
- 2 eggs, beaten

- 1/2 tsp onion powder
- 1/4 cup sunflower seeds, crushed
- 1/2 cup almond flour
- 1 tsp salt

Directions:

1. Preheat the oven to 450 F.
2. In a bowl, add beaten eggs.
3. In another bowl, add almond flour, sunflower seed, onion powder, and salt.
4. Dip avocado slices in egg mixture then coat with almond flour mixture and place on baking sheet.
5. Bake in preheated oven for 20 minutes.
6. Serve and enjoy.

Nutrition Value:

Calories 274

Fat 25 g

Carbs 10 g

Sugar 1 g

Protein 6 g

Cholesterol 82 mg

59. Baked Onion Rings

Preparation Time: 35 minutes

Servings: 4

Ingredients:

- 2 eggs
- 2 large onion, chopped into rings
- 1/2 tsp black pepper
- 1/2 tsp garlic powder
- 2 tbsp thyme, sliced
- 1 1/2 cups almond flour

- 1/2 tsp salt

Directions:

1. Preheat the oven to 400 F.
2. In a bowl, whisk eggs.
3. In another bowl, combine together almond flour, thyme, salt, garlic powder, and black pepper.
4. Dip onion rings in egg mixture then coat with almond flour mixture and place on baking sheet.
5. Bake in preheated oven for 25 minutes.
6. Serve hot and enjoy.

Nutrition Value:

Calories 127

Fat 7 g

Carbs 10 g

Sugar 4 g

Protein 6 g

Cholesterol 82 mg

60. Easy Brussels sprouts Chips

Preparation Time: 15 minutes

Servings: 2

Ingredients:

- 10 Brussels sprouts split leaves
- 1 tbsp extra virgin olive oil
- 1/4 tsp salt

Directions:

1. Preheat the oven to 350 F.
2. Add all ingredients to the bowl and toss well.
3. Place Brussels sprouts on baking sheet and roast in preheated oven for 10 minutes.
4. Serve and enjoy.

Nutrition Value:

Calories 101

Fat 7 g

Carbs 8 g

Sugar 2 g

Protein 3 g

Cholesterol 0 mg

61. Crispy Apple Chips

Preparation Time: 2 hours 5 minutes

Servings: 6

Ingredients:

- 2 medium apples, cored and sliced
- 2 tbsp pumpkin pie spice
- Directions:
- Preheat the oven to 390 F.

- Arrange apple slices on a baking sheet.
- Sprinkle pumpkin pie spice on apple slices and bake in preheated oven for 2 hours.
- Serve and enjoy.

Nutrition Value:

Calories 45

Fat 0.4 g

Carbs 11 g

Sugar 7 g

Protein 0.3 g

Cholesterol 0 mg

62. Zucchini Chips

Preparation Time: 25 minutes

Servings: 3

Ingredients:

- 4 small zucchinis, sliced

- 1/2 cup parmesan cheese, grated
- Pepper
- Salt

Directions:

1. Arrange sliced zucchinis on a baking sheet.
2. Sprinkle parmesan cheese over sliced zucchinis.
3. Season with pepper and salt.
4. Bake at 425 F for 15 minutes.
5. Serve hot and enjoy.

Nutrition Value:

Calories 45

Fat 2 g

Carbs 5 g

Sugar 2 g

Protein 4 g

Cholesterol 4 mg

63. Crisp Radish Chips

Preparation Time: 25 minutes

Servings: 4

Ingredients:

1. 16 oz fresh radishes
2. 2 tbsp olive oil
3. 1/2 tsp pepper
4. 1/2 tsp sea salt

Directions:

- Preheat the oven to 400 F.
- Add all ingredients to the bowl and toss well.
- Arrange sliced radishes on a baking sheet and bake in preheated oven for 15 minutes.
- Serve and enjoy.

Nutrition Value:

Calories 79

Fat 7 g

Carbs 4 g

Sugar 2 g

Protein 0.8 g

Cholesterol 0 mg

64. Fried Parsnip Chips

Preparation Time: 15 minutes

Servings: 4

Ingredients:

- 2 medium parsnips, peeled and sliced
- Salt
- Oil for frying

Directions:

- Heat oil in a large saucepan over medium-high

heat.

- Once the oil temperature reaches 350 F then add sliced parsnips into the batches in oil and fry for 30 seconds or until lightly golden brown.

- Place fried parsnips chips on a paper towel to soak extra oil.

- Sprinkle salt over fried parsnip chips and serve.

Nutrition Value:

Calories 50

Fat 2 g

Carbs 12 g

Sugar 3.2 g

Protein 0.8 g

Cholesterol 0 mg

65. Spicy Roasted Nuts

Preparation Time: 30 minutes

Servings: 4

Ingredients:

- 1/2 cup almonds
- 1/2 cup walnuts
- 1/2 cup hazelnuts
- 1 tsp cinnamon
- 1 tsp ginger root
- 1 tsp fresh orange peel
- 1 tsp nutmeg
- 4 tbsp olive oil
- 1 tsp sea salt

Directions:

1. Preheat the oven to 375 F.
2. Add almonds, walnuts, and hazelnuts in a bowl and toss well.

3. Place nuts on a baking sheet and roast in preheated oven for 10 minutes.
4. Melt butter in a pan over medium heat.
5. Once butter is melted then add cinnamon, ginger root, orange peel, nutmeg, and salt in a pan and stir well.
6. Add roasted nuts in a pan and toss well.
7. Serve hot and enjoy.

Nutrition Value:
Calories 349

Fat 35 g

Carbs 6 g

Sugar 1 g

Protein 7 g

Cholesterol 0 mg

SOUPS AND SALADS

66. Greek-Style Salad

Preparation Time: 3 hours 15 minutes

Servings 4

Nutrition Value: 208 Calories; 15.6g Fat; 6.2g Carbs; 7.6g Protein; 5.1G Fiber

Ingredients

For Sunflower Seed Dressing:

- 1 cup sunflower seeds, raw and hulled
- 2 cups of water
- 2 tablespoons scallions, chopped
- 1 garlic clove, chopped
- 1 lime, freshly squeezed
- Salt and black pepper, to taste
- 1/2 teaspoon red pepper flakes crushed
- 1/4 teaspoon rosemary, minced

- 2 tablespoons coconut milk

For the salad:

- 1 fresh head lettuce, separated into leaves
- 3 tomatoes, diced
- 3 cucumbers, sliced
- 2 tablespoons Kalamata olives, pitted

Directions

1. Soak the sunflower seeds in water at least 3 hours.Drain the sunflower seeds; transfer them to your blender and add the remaining ingredients for the dressing.
2. Puree until creamy, smooth and uniform.
3. Put all the salad ingredients into four serving bowls. Toss with the dressing and serve immediately. Bon appétit!

67. Moroccan Carrot Salad With Harissa

Preparation Time: 10 minutes

Servings 4

Nutrition Value: 196 Calories; 17.2G Fat; 6g Carbs; 1.2G Protein; 3.5g Fiber

Ingredients

- 1 pound carrots, coarsely shredded
- 1/4 cup fresh cilantro,chopped
- For the Vinaigrette:
- 3 garlic cloves, smashed
- Sea salt and ground black pepper, to taste
- 1/3 cup extra-virgin olive oil
- 1 lime, freshly squeezed
- 2 tablespoons balsamic vinegar
- 1/2 teaspoon ground cumin
- 1/2 teaspoon harissa

Directions

1. Place the shredded carrots and fresh, chopped cilantro in a salad bowl.
2. Combine all ingredients for the vinaigrette; mix until everything is well incorporated.
3. Add the vinaigrette to the carrot salad and toss to coat well. Bon appétit!

68. Warm Savoy Cabbage Slaw

Preparation Time: 25 minutes

Servings 4

Nutrition Value: 118 Calories; 7g Fat; 6.7g Carbs; 2.9g Protein; 5g Fiber

Ingredients

- 2 pounds Savoy cabbage, torn into pieces
- 2 tablespoons almond oil
- 1 teaspoon garlic, minced
- 1/2 teaspoon dried basil

- 1/2 teaspoon red pepper flakes, crushed
- Salt and ground black pepper, to the taste

Directions

1. Cook the Savoy cabbage in a pot of a lightly salted water approximately 20 minutes over moderate heat. Drain and reserve.
2. Now, heat the oil in a sauté pan over medium-high heat. Now, cook the garlic until just aromatic.
3. Add the reserved Savoy cabbage, basil, red pepper, salt, and black pepper; stir until everything is heated through.
4. Taste, adjust the seasonings, and serve warm over cauliflower rice.

69. Taco Salad Boats

Preparation Time: 25 minutes

Servings 4

Nutrition Value: 140 Calories; 10.8g Fat; 7.2G

Carbs; 4.3g Protein; 5g Fiber

Ingredients

- 1 head romaine lettuce, stems removed
- 1/2 cup canned black beans
- 1 cup tomatoes, chopped
- 1 medium bunch of scallions, sliced
- 2 peppers, shredded
- 1 cup red cabbage, shredded
- 1 ripe avocado, peeled, pitted and diced
- 1/2 cup sesame butter
- 1 tablespoon apple cider vinegar
- 1 tablespoon fresh lime juice
- 1 teaspoon chili powder
- Sea salt and ground black pepper, to taste
- 1/2 red pepper flakes

Directions

1. Pull the leaves off of the romaine hearts and arrange them on a tray.

2. In a mixing bowl, combine the black beans with the tomatoes, scallions, peppers, red cabbage, and avocado. Fill the romaine “boats” with the bean mixture.

3. Then, mix the sesame butter with the apple cider vinegar, lime juice, chili powder, salt, and black pepper. Drizzle the sauce over the filling.

4. Garnish with red pepper flakes and serve immediately. Bon appétit!

70. Cauliflower Salad With Pecans

Preparation Time: 15 minutes + chilling time

Servings 4

Nutrition Value: 281 Calories; 26.8g Fat; 5.6g Carbs; 4.2G Protein; 3.8g Fiber

Ingredients

- 1 head fresh cauliflower, cut into florets
- 1 cup spring onions, chopped
- 4 ounces bottled roasted peppers, chopped
- 1/4 cup extra-virgin olive oil
- 1 tablespoon wine vinegar
- 1 teaspoon yellow mustard
- Coarse salt and black pepper, to your liking
- 1/2 cup green olives, pitted and chopped
- 1/2 cup pecans, coarsely chopped

Directions

1. Steam the cauliflower florets for 4 to 6 minutes; set aside to cool.
2. In a salad bowl, place the spring onions and roasted peppers.
3. In a mixing dish, whisk the olive oil, vinegar,

mustard, salt, and pepper. Drizzle over the veggies in the salad bowl.

4. Now, add the reserved cauliflower and toss to combine well. Scatter the green olives and pecans over the top and serve.

71. Crunchy Broccoli Salad

Preparation Time: 5 minutes + chilling time

Servings 4

Nutrition Value: 245 Calories; 22.8g Fat; 6g Carbs; 4.2G Protein; 4.3g Fiber

Ingredients

- 1 pound frozen broccoli, thawed and broken into small florets
- 1 cup green onions, chopped
- 1 bell pepper, sliced
- 1/4 cup pecan, slivered
- 1/3 cup extra-virgin olive oil

- 2 tablespoons balsamic vinegar
- 1/2 teaspoon basil
- 1/2 teaspoon oregano
- Sea salt and freshly ground black pepper

Directions

1. Thoroughly combine all ingredients in a salad bowl.
2. Cover and let it sit in your refrigerator until ready to serve. Bon appétit!

72. Kale Salad With Crispy Tofu Cubes

Preparation Time: 15 minutes

Servings 4

Nutrition Value: 327 Calories; 29.1G Fat; 7.2G Carbs; 13.2G Protein; 3.7g Fiber

Ingredients

- 2 tablespoons coconut oil

- 1 (14-ounce) block extra-firm tofu, pressed and cubed
- 1 bunch kale, torn into small pieces
- 1 shallot, sliced
- 1 garlic clove, pressed
- 1/4 cup cilantro leaves, divided
- 1 jalapeno pepper, seeded and minced
- 1/4 cup olive oil
- 1 lemon, juices
- Sea salt and ground black pepper, to taste
- 1 (1-inch) piece fresh ginger, peeled and grated
- 1 tablespoon coconut aminos
- 1 tablespoon sunflower seeds, lightly toasted
- 1 tablespoon pumpkin seeds, lightly toasted

Directions

1. Heat the coconut oil in a saucepan over medium heat; now, cook the tofu cubes until they are golden brown on all sides. Reserve.
2. Mix the kale, shallot, garlic, cilantro, and jalapeno pepper in a salad bowl; then, drizzle the salad with olive oil and lemon juice.
3. Add the salt, pepper, ginger, and coconut aminos; toss to combine well. Top with the reserved tofu cubes. Scatter lightly toasted seeds over your salad and serve.

73. Cucumber And Zucchini Ribbon Salad

Preparation Time: 15 minutes

Servings 4

Nutrition Value: 252 Calories; 23.1G Fat; 6.1G Carbs; 3.5g Protein; 2.7g Fiber

Ingredients

- 2 medium cucumbers, julienned

- 2 medium zucchinis, julienned
- 1 teaspoon of sea salt
- 2 tomatoes, sliced
- 1 WHIte onion, chopped
- 1 cup rocket lettuce, torn into pieces
- 1/3 cup extra-virgin olive oil
- 1 teaspoon fresh garlic, pressed
- 2 tablespoons balsamic vinegar
- 1 tablespoon Dijon mustard
- Sea salt and ground black pepper, to taste
- 2 tablespoons sesame seeds, lightly toasted
- 2 tablespoons sunflower seeds, lightly toasted

Directions

1. Toss the cucumber and zucchini with 1 teaspoon of sea salt in a fine-mesh sieve; place

the sieve over the bowl.

2. Let it sit for about 20 minutes; then, squeeze the cucumber and zucchini gently to remove any excess liquid. Transfer them to a large bowl.

3. Add in the tomatoes, onion, and rocket lettuce. Make the vinaigrette by whisking the olive oil, garlic, balsamic vinegar, mustard, salt, and black pepper to taste.

4. Dress your salad and serve garnished with lightly toasted seeds. Eat immediately or place in your refrigerator until ready to serve!

74. Crazy Asian Zucchini Salad:

Servings: 10

Preparation Time: 10 to 15minutes

Nutrition Value:

Calories: 120

Protein: 4g

Fat: 1G

Carbs: 7.3g

Ingredients:

- 1 lb. Cabbage (shredded
- 1/3 cup White vinegar
- 1 cup Sunflower seeds (shelled)
- 1 cup Almonds (sliced)
- 1 ½ teaspoon Stevia drops – about
- ¾ cup Avocado oil
- 1 Zucchini (thinly spiralized)

Direction:

- First of all, please check that you've all the ingredients on the market. Toss together the cabbage, zucchini, almonds & sunflower seeds in a bowl.
- Now whisk together the vinegar, oil & stevia in

a bowl.

- One thing remains to be done. Add the dressing to the salad & toss.
- Finally, refrigerate for about 2 hours.

75. Iconic Creamy Kale Salad:

Servings: 3

Preparation Time: 20 to 30 minutes

Nutrition Value:

Calories: 78

Protein: 1.1 g

Fat: 6.4 g

Carbs: 3.2 g

Ingredients:

a) 1 bunch spinach

b) 1 ½ tablespoon lemon juice

c) 1 cup sour cream

d) 1 cup roasted macadamia

e) 2 tablespoons sesame seeds oil

f) ½ cup parmesan cheese, grated

g) 1 ½ garlic clove, minced

h) ½ teaspoon black pepper

i) ¼ teaspoon salt

j) 2 tablespoons lime juice

k) 1 bunch kale

Toppings:

l) 1 ½ Avocado, diced

m) 1/4 cup Pecans, chopped

n) 3 oz. Goat cheese

Direction:

1. First of all, please confirm you've all the ingredients out there. Chop kale and wash kale then remove the ribs.

2. Now transfer kale to a large bowl.
3. One thing remains to be done. Add sour cream, lime juice, macadamia, sesame seeds oil, pepper, salt, garlic, and grated cheese.
4. Finally, mix thoroughly. Top with your avocado, goat cheese, and pecans. Serve& enjoy.

76. Tasty Corn & Avocado Salad

Servings: 4

Preparation Time: 4 to 5 minutes

Nutrition Value:

Calories: 144

Protein: 3.2 g

Fat: 13 g

Carbs: 8 g

Ingredients:

Salad:

- 1 Corn on the cob(cooked, cut off husk)
- 4 ½ Grape tomatoes(quartered)
- ¼ cup Red onions (sliced)
- 1 Romaine head (chopped)
- ½ Avocado(sliced)

Dressing:

- Just a pinch Black pepper
- 1 ½ tablespoon Shallots(minced)
- 2 tablespoons White wine vinegar
- ½ teaspoon Kosher salt
- 6 tablespoons buttermilk
- 2 tablespoons Dijon mustard
- ¼ teaspoon Garlic powder

- 2 tablespoons virgin olive oil

Direction:

1. First of all, active and assemble all the ingredients in one place. Now for the dressing, whisk together all the dressing, whisk together all the dressing ingredients.
2. Finally, combine all the salad ingredients in a bowl along with the dressing & toss together. Finally, we've completed the recipe. Enjoy.

77. Coolest Arugula & Blueberry Salad:

Servings: 6 to 7

Preparation Time: 5 to 10minutes

Nutrition Value:

Calories: 121

Protein: 6 g

Fat: 13 g

Carbs: 5 g

Ingredients:

- 2 cups Blueberries
- 2 ½ tablespoons Balsamic vinegar
- 1 tablespoon Dijon mustard
- 10 oz. Arugula
- 2 ½ tablespoons Fresh orange juice
- ¼ cup Avocado oil

Direction:

1. First of all, ahead and assemble all the ingredients in one place. Now toss together the blueberries & arugula in a bowl.

2. Only one thing remains to be done now. Whisk along the remainder of the ingredients in another bowl.

3. Finally, pour the dressing over the dish and toss. Finally, we've completed the recipe. Enjoy.

78. Fantastic Clean Avocado Salad with Cilantro:

Servings: 4 to 6

Preparation Time: 10 to 15MINutes

Nutrition Value:

Calories: 126

Protein: 2.1G

Fat: 10g

Carbs: 10g

Ingredients:

- 1 chopped up a sweet
- Pepper as needed
- green bell pepper(chopped up)
- 1 large sized chopped up red tomato
- Salt as needed
- ¼ cup of chopped up fresh cilantro

- avocados peeled, pitted and diced
- ½ of a juiced

Direction:

1. First of all, please confirm you've all the ingredients obtainable. Take a medium-sized bowl and add onions, bell pepper, tomato, avocados, cilantro& lime juice
2. Then mix well & coat everything well
3. One thing remains to be done. Season with some salt & pepper
4. Finally, serve chilled!

79. Curious Courgette Salad with Herbed Vinaigrette:

Servings: 4 to 5

Preparation Time: 20 to 25 minutes

Nutrition Value:

Calories: 76

Protein: 2.1 g

Fat: 4.1 g

Carbs: 3.1 g

Ingredients:

- 2 ½ tablespoons Olive oil
- Salt and pepper to taste
- ½ pack Chopped chives
- 1 lemon juice
- 1 pack Chopped mint
- 10 ½ oz. Courgettes (spiralized using the large noodle attachment of the spiralizer)

Direction:

- First of all, go ahead and assemble all the ingredients in one place. Combine the salt, lemon juice, pepper and olive oil in a bowl and whisk together.

- Mix in the herbs.
- Combine the courgette noodles & the dressing in a bowl and toss together. Finally, we've completed the recipe. Enjoy.

80. Keto Red Curry

Servings: 6-8

Preparation Time: About 40 minutes

Ingredients:

- 1 cup broccoli florets
- 1 large handful of fresh spinach
- 4 Tbsp. coconut oil
- ¼ medium onion
- 1 tsp. garlic, minced
- 1 tsp. fresh ginger, peeled and minced
- 2 tsp. soy sauce
- 1 Tbsp. red curry paste

- ½ cup coconut cream

Directions:

- Add half the coconut oil to a saucepan and heat over medium-high heat.
- When the oil is hot, add the onion to the pan and saute for 3-4 minutes, until it is semi-translucent. Add the garlic to the pan and saute, stirring, just until fragrant, about 30 seconds.
- Lower the heat to medium-low and add broccoli florets. Saute, stirring, for about 1-2 minutes.
- Push the vegetables to the side of the pan and add the red curry paste. Saute until the paste is fragrant, then mix everything together.
- Add the spinach on top of the vegetable mixture. When the spinach begins to wilt, add the coconut cream and stir.

- Add the rest of the coconut oil, the soy sauce, and the minced ginger. Bring to a simmer for 5-10 minutes.
- Serve hot.

Nutrition Value:

Total Fat: 41 g

Carbs: 8 g

Protein: 4 g

81. Kale Soup

Servings: 6-8

Preparation Time:About 40 minutes

Ingredients:

- 4 cups fresh kale, chopped
- ½ cup canned white beans
- 2 cloves garlic, minced
- ½ onion, diced

- ½ cup celery, diced
- ¼ tsp. freshly ground black pepper
- Salt to taste
- 1 cup of water

Directions:

1. Place all ingredients into a heavy stockpot.
2. Bring to a low simmer and cook until fragrant, about 30 minutes. Add water if necessary during cooking.
3. Transfer the soup to serving bowls and serve hot.

Nutrition Value:

Total Fat: 15 g

Carbs: 15 g

Protein: 9 g

82. Creamy Jalapeno Soup

Servings: 8-10

Preparation Time: About 45 minutes

Ingredients:

- 3 Tbsp. butter
- 2 cloves garlic, minced
- ½ onion, chopped
- ½ bell pepper, chopped
- 2 jalapeno peppers, seeded and chopped
- 6 oz. cream cheese
- 3 cups vegetable stock
- ½ cup heavy cream
- ¼ tsp. paprika
- 1 tsp. cumin
- 1 tsp. salt
- ½ tsp. freshly ground black pepper

Directions:

1. Heat the oil in a heavy stockpot over medium-high heat. When the butter is melted, add onion, bell pepper, and jalapenos and sauté until the onion is soft about 5 minutes.
2. Add the stock and
3. cream cheese to the pot, stirring to combine.
4. Bring to a low simmer and cook until the chicken is thoroughly cooked and the vegetables are tender about 30 minutes. Add water if necessary during cooking.
5. Stir in the cream, stirring to combine.
6. Transfer to serving bowls and serve hot topped with grated cheese.

Nutrition Value:

Total Fat: 40 g

Carbs: 4 g

Protein: 41 g

83. Chinese Chili Soup

Servings: 8-10

Preparation Time: About 40 minutes

Ingredients:

- ¼ cup sesame oil
- 6 dried red Thai chilis
- 5 cloves garlic, crushed
- 2 Tbsp. fresh ginger, peeled and sliced
- 3 cups vegetable stock
- ¼ cup of soy sauce
- ¼ cup dry sherry
- Salt to taste
- ¼ cup fresh Thai basil, chopped

Directions:

1. Heat the oil in a heavy stockpot over medium-high heat. Add the garlic, chilis, and ginger to

the pot and sauté just until fragrant, about a minute.

2. Lower the heat and add all the other ingredients, excluding the basil, to the pot.
3. Bring to a low simmer and cook until the soup is fragrant about 30 minutes. Add water if necessary during cooking.
4. Bring the soup to a boil again and stir in the basil, stirring until the basil is fragrant and wilted.
5. Transfer to serving bowls and serve hot.

Nutrition Value:

Total Fat: 15 g

Carbs: 7 g

Protein: 31 g

84. Mushroom Soup

Servings: 8-10

Preparation Time: About 40 minutes

Ingredients:

- 1 onion, chopped
- 3 cloves garlic, minced
- 2 cups fresh button mushrooms, chopped
- 1 medium yellow summer squash, chopped
- 3 cups vegetable stock
- Salt and pepper to taste
- 1 tsp. poultry seasoning

Directions:

1. Add all ingredients to a heavy stockpot.
2. Bring to a low simmer and cook until the soup is fragrant about 30 minutes. Add water if necessary during cooking.
3. Transfer soup to serving bowls and serve hot.

Nutrition Value:

Total Fat: 15 g

Carbs: 9 g

Protein: 30 g

85. Vietnamese-Style Vegetable Soup

Servings: 6-8

Preparation Time: About 40 minutes

Ingredients:

- 1 onion, diced
- 2 Tbsp. tomato paste
- 2 whole star anise
- 1 Tbsp. fresh ginger, peeled and minced
- 3 cloves garlic, minced
- 6 cups of water
- 1 tsp. ground pepper

- ½ tsp. Chinese five-spice
- ½ tsp. curry powder
- 2 carrots, peeled and sliced

Directions:

1. Place all ingredients in a heavy stockpot.
2. Bring to a low simmer and cook until the soup is fragrant about 30 minutes. Add water if necessary during cooking.
3. Serve the stew hot.

Nutrition Value:

Total Fat: 9 g

Carbs: 8 g

Protein: 15 g

86. Green Chili Soup

Servings: 6-8

Preparation Time: About 2 hours

Ingredients:

- ½ cup dry navy beans, soaked for an hour in hot water
- 1 onion diced
- 3 New Mexico green chili peppers, chopped
- 5 cloves garlic, minced
- 1 cup cauliflower, diced
- 4 cups vegetable stock
- ¼ cup fresh cilantro, chopped
- 1 tsp. ground coriander
- 1 tsp. ground cumin
- 1 tsp. salt
- 2 oz. cream cheese

Directions:

1. Put all the ingredients, excluding the cream cheese, into a large, heavy stockpot.

2. Bring to a low simmer and cook until the beans are tender about 60 minutes. Add water if necessary during cooking.

3. Using an immersion blender, blend the soup until it is smooth.

4. Return the soup to a simmer.

5. When the soup is bubbly, stir in the cream cheese until it's melted.

6. Transfer the soup to serving bowls and serve hot.

Nutrition Value:

Total Fat: 5 g

Carbs: 13 g

Protein: 22 g

87. Vegetarian Red Chili

Servings: 6-8

Preparation Time: About 35 minutes

Ingredients:

- 3 tsp. chili powder
- 2 tsp. ground cumin
- 2 tsp. salt
- 1 tsp. dried oregano
- 1 Tbsp. olive oil
- 1 onion, chopped
- 2 cloves garlic, minced
- 1 cup canned diced tomatoes
- 1 Tbsp. canned chipotle chilis, chopped
- 2 corn tortillas, torn into small pieces
- ½ cup of water

Directions:

1. In a small bowl, mix chili powder, cumin, salt, and oregano.

2. In a blender or food processor, blend tomatoes, chilis, and tortilla pieces until smooth.

3. Heat the oil in a heavy stockpot over medium-high heat. When the oil is hot, sauté the onions until they're softened, about 3 minutes. Add the garlic and sauté for about a minute more.

4. Stir in the spice mixture and sauté until fragrant, about 30 seconds.

5. Add the tomato/tortilla mixture to the pot, along with 2 cups water.

6. Bring to a low simmer and cook until fragrant about 20 minutes. Add water if necessary during cooking.

7. Transfer the chili to serving bowls and serve hot.

Nutrition Value:
Total Fat: 24 g

Carbs: 12 g

Protein: 30 g

88. Vegetarian Green Chili

Servings: 6-8

Preparation Time: About 30 minutes

Ingredients:

- 3 tomatillos, sliced
- 3 jalapeno peppers, seeded and chopped
- 2 New Mexico green chili peppers, seeded and chopped
- 6 cloves garlic, minced
- 1 tomato, chopped
- 3 cups vegetable stock
- 2 tsp. cumin
- Salt and pepper to taste

Directions:

1. Put the tomatillos, jalapenos, New Mexico

chilis, garlic, chicken stock, and tomato into a heavy stockpot.

2. Add the cumin, salt, and pepper on top of the meat.
3. Bring to a low simmer and cook until fragrant, about 20 minutes. Add water if necessary during cooking.
4. Using an immersion blender, blend the sauce in the pot until it's smooth.
5. Transfer the chili to serving bowls and serve hot, garnished with chopped fresh cilantro.

Nutrition Value:
Total Fat: 4 g

Carbs: 4 g

Protein: 26 g

89. Tortilla Soup

Servings: 6-8

Preparation Time: About 30 minutes

Ingredients:

1. 2 corn tortillas, torn into pieces
2. ½ onion, chopped
3. 1 cup tomatoes, chopped
4. 2 cloves garlic
5. 1 Tbsp. canned chipotle chili in adobo sauce, chopped
6. ½ jalapeno pepper
7. ¼ cup fresh cilantro, chopped
8. 1 tsp. salt
9. 1 Tbsp. olive oil
10. 4 cups of water

Directions:

1. In a blender or food processor, combine onion, tomatoes, garlic, chipotle, jalapeno, and

cilantro. Blend until the mixture is smooth.

2. Heat the oil in a heavy stockpot over medium-high heat. When the oil is hot, add the blended mixture to the pot. Cook, stirring, until fragrant, about a minute or two.

3. Add the tortillas, chicken, and water to the pot.

4. Bring to a low simmer and cook until fragrant, about 20 minutes. Add water if necessary during cooking.

5. Transfer to serving bowls and serve hot.

Nutrition Value:

Total Fat: 5 g

Carbs: 5 g

Protein: 12 g

90. Keto Vegetable Soup

Servings: 6-8

Preparation Time: About 45 minutes

Ingredients:

- 1 turnip, cut into bite-size pieces
- 1 onion, chopped
- 6 stalks celery, diced
- 1 carrot, sliced
- 15 oz. pumpkin puree
- 1 lb. green beans frozen or fresh
- 8 cups chicken stock
- 2 cups of water
- 1 Tbsp. fresh basil, chopped
- ¼ tsp. thyme leaves
- 1/8 tsp. rubbed sage
- Salt to taste
- 1 lb. fresh spinach, chopped

Directions:

1. Put all the ingredients, excluding the spinach, into a heavy stockpot.
2. Bring to a low simmer and cook until the vegetables are tender about 30 minutes. Add water if necessary during cooking.
3. Add the spinach and stir until it's wilted about 5 minutes.
4. Transfer to serving bowls and serve hot.

Nutrition Value:

Total Fat: 0 gram

Carbs: 10 g

Protein: 3 g

91. Keto Cabbage Soup

Servings: 6-8

Preparation Time: About 45 minutes

Ingredients:

- ¼ cup onion, diced
- 1 clove garlic, minced
- 1 tsp. cumin
- 1 head cabbage, chopped
- 1 ¼ cup canned diced tomatoes
- 5 oz. canned green chilis
- 4 cups vegetable stock
- Salt and pepper to taste

Directions:

1. Heat a heavy stockpot over medium-high heat. When the oil is hot, add the onions and sauté for 5-7 minutes more. Add the garlic and sauté for one more minute.

2. Bring to a low simmer and cook until the vegetables are tender about 30 minutes. Add water if necessary, during cooking.

3. Transfer to serving bowls and serve hot.

Nutrition Value:

Total Fat: 18 g

Carbs: 6 g

Protein: 17 g

CONCLUSION

I hope this keto vegan guide has helped you learn that vegan can be super tasty and why we need to save our animals and our planet and most of all, why the vegan diet is just what you need to steer your health in the right direction.

The next step is to jump right into the diet by making healthy and smart vegan food choices to ensure you meet your recommended daily nutrition. If you are starting out on veganism, you should join an online vegan group that will further guide you on the best way to take up the vegan diet and tips and tricks to stay on a diet.

We have seen the immense health benefits of the vegan diet. Combine it with regular exercise, clean water, and healthy habits, and you will discover the fountain of health and youth.

CPSIA information can be obtained
at www.ICGtesting.com
Printed in the USA
LVHW021934240121
677375LV00028B/918

9 781801 58232